fasting

A WAY TO WELL-BEING

Judith H. Dobrzynski

SOVEREIGN BOOKS
NEW YORK

We strongly recommend that anyone considering fasting first consult a physician before engaging in a fast.

Published by Sovereign Books
A Simon & Schuster Division of
Gulf & Western Corporation
Simon & Schuster Building
1230 Avenue of the Americas
New York, New York 10020
Designed by Libra Graphics, Inc.
Manufactured in the United States of America
10 9 8 7 6 5 4 3 2 1
Library of Congress Cataloging in Publication Data
Dobrzynski, Judith H
Fasting.
Bibliography: p.
Includes index.
1. Fasting. I. Title.
RM226.D62 394.1'2 78-26063
ISBN 0-671-18408-3
ISBN 0-671-18355-9 pbk.

contents

foreword vii

1 in the midst of plenty 1

2 why fasting is blossoming 7

3 origin and folklore 17

4 religious traditions 25

5 political fasts 43

6 to your health? 53

7 the surest way to lose weight 69

8 how the body adjusts to a fast 83

9 how to fast 95

10 fasting farms 105

epilog 109

bibliography 113

index 117

foreword

JUDITH DOBRZYNSKI's book on fasting is the best guide to sensible eating I have ever read. It appealed to me in three ways:

- As a formerly fat person who must fast in order to maintain a healthy and attractive body, I found her review of this method of weight control both enlightening and reassuring.
- As a medical doctor who cringes each time a patient asks me about a new fad diet, I sighed with relief upon reading this author's clear review of how people lose weight *on any diet*. Ms. Dobrzynski cuts through much of the nonsense, confusion, and mystery surrounding weight loss. The reader will find a clear and simple path toward good nutrition, devoid of hocus-pocus, plus common-sense information on sound dietary practices.
- As a psychiatrist, I consider eating the oldest addiction of mankind. So powerful is this desire that we are unable to change entrenched eating patterns, even to save our lives. Fasting, the author reveals, helps cure our addiction to unnecessary food, revives our senses, and guides us to sounder nutritional habits.

The body is a system for manufacturing energy. Like every other system or machine, it requires periods of rest. By giving the body a chemical holiday (that is, by fasting), we allow the digestive and excretory mechanisms to be renewed.

Americans are growing increasingly health conscious. People who considered themselves put out to pasture years ago are now jogging three miles around the pasture each day. Many of us are convinced that nutritional salvation awaits us if only we leave the crowded supermarket aisles and hasten to our local health food stores, which stock vitamins, granola, and longevity in metrically measured packages. One of the strongest features of this book is the author's treatment of competing claims made by nutritional advocates of every stripe. She reviews the most important controversies about fasting, dieting, and nutrition in general, and provides clear assessments of their relative merits. In addition, she makes us see the logic of sound nutrition without making outlandish claims for any method. From this information, the reader can make judgments about which camp, if any, to join.

I found Ms. Dobrzynski's discussion of Dick Gregory's experiences fascinating. For him, fasting began as a political protest and only later became a valuable health practice. Long forgotten and dulled senses were revived during his fasts and he found himself able to think more clearly. The biological result was that his body developed the ability to discriminate—no longer could he tolerate junk food. Just as inane television programs dull our senses, a steady diet of garbage foods dulls our bodies' natural instincts until they can no longer reject deficient and harmful elements. Fasting helps these instincts remain acute.

Fasting helps us rediscover what good food really tastes like. I experienced this personally during my own weight-control struggle. I finally realized that I would always psychologically be a fat person. I know I will always love eating. Like a heroin addict, I need my "fix" just to feel normal, but too much food dulls my appreciation. Now I know that to really enjoy a feast, I should fast beforehand.

One of the most appealing aspects of this book is the author's review of the history and religious uses of fasts. Fasting, as she points out, widespread elsewhere, is growing among Americans. This practice is not threatening, provided you know its effects on your body. The author gives guidance about the precautions you should take during a fast, the bodily sensations you will feel, and the way you should reenter the eating process. For those who like assistance, concise evaluations of some well-known fasting farms are provided.

For people who want to reshape their eating habits and/or their bodies, *Fasting* is the most readable and useful book available to date on eating or not eating, and remaining healthy either way.

SIDNEY LECKER, M.D.

1
in the midst of plenty

"There is no love sincerer than the love of food," wrote George Bernard Shaw. Americans believe him. We love our food. We hunger for other earthly delights, too, but often not as passionately. The way other nationalities love wine, or music, or the sea, Americans savor and enjoy their food. Of course, other nations have a tradition of food appreciation; the French, for example, are famous for their meals. So are the Italians, the Greeks, the Chinese. But somehow America's love affair with food runs deeper. Here food is rarely considered to be strictly utilitarian, something necessary for life but not meant to be enjoyed in and of itself. For many reasons—among them the country's youth, immigrant roots, fast living pace, and wealth—Americans display a deep, catholic, almost indiscriminating love of food. Fast food, health food, high-protein, high-fat red meats, ethnic dishes, junk food, and good old American apple pie (a la mode, if possible)—we love it all. Family and social life often centers around food. A full stomach means that, for the moment at least, all is well.

Lately, in fact, interest in food in the United States has been stronger than ever. Each year we're eating more than we had been. The trend toward more varied menus for American breakfasts, brunches, lunches, suppers, dinners, and bedtime snacks recently has risen like a cheese soufflé. Cookbooks are selling, pardon the expression, faster than hotcakes. And they are much more specialized than those of the past; publishers are making millions on sales of entire books about herb cookery, cheese dishes, blender cooking, yogurt-based recipes, regional specialties, even junk foods. Yes, Americans are paying more attention to the details of their food. Sales of kitchen gadgets have skyrocketed, too; retailers sometimes have trouble keeping shelves stocked with peanut butter machines, tortilla presses, woks, vegetable steamers, ice cream makers, melon-ballers, and other items you didn't think even had names.

Our rapidly changing lifestyle influences our eating habits, and many factors have changed vastly over the last century—we have more mobility, more divorces, more single people, more working mothers, more convenience foods, more automobiles, more disposable income, more knowledge, and more foods from which to choose. The Department of Agriculture says each of us now eats about 1,900 pounds of food each year—more than five pounds a day. USDA also says we eat an average of 3,300 calories of food each day. We spend $215 billion each year on food in the supermarket and in restaurants—about $1,000 for each man, woman, and child. Food is relatively more expensive in most other parts of the world, so Americans spend less on, but eat more, food than any other country for which the government collects statistics. The French, for example, eat an average of about 2,850 calories a day; the Japanese consume only a few more than 1,900 calories each day.

We also care more about the food we eat than we used to. In 1976, the Gallup poll organization asked Americans about nutrition, and found that 88 percent of us wanted to know more about it. A year later, a Harris poll discovered that only "fourteen percent of those questioned thought Americans ate a proper diet." We not only love food, we don't think we are all eating as well as we could be and we want to know more about how we can.

So then, it might seem paradoxical to note that in the midst of all this preoccupation with food, many Americans and many citizens of other countries voluntarily fast—go entirely without food—for a day or days at a time. Fasting, in fact, has been gaining popularity over the last ten or fifteen years.

Fasting has been around for centuries, since prehistoric times.

Archaeologists have found ancient tablets mentioning it. The Bible talks about fasting on about seventy-five occasions. Socrates and Plato and Pythagoras did it to prepare for tests of their intellectual powers. Shakespeare weaves fasting into the blank verse of *Hamlet, The Merchant of Venice,* and at least three other plays. Franz Kafka wrote a short story about it, "The Hunger Artist," published in 1924. Today's chronicles carry articles about fasting and fasters, too. According to recent stories in newspapers and magazines, the panoply of celebrities who fast now or have fasted includes California Governor Edmund G. (Jerry) Brown, Jr., actresses Cloris Leachman, Jane Fonda, Shirley MacLaine, and Valerie Harper, basketball player Bill Walton, writers Norman Mailer and Pete Hammill, Senator Mark Hatfield, all-American-girl model Cheryl Tiegs, and consumerist Lola Redford, Robert's wife. Others might try it if they took a good look at another famous faster, that ageless grandfather, Pat Boone.

Yet, for all this publicity, not many people understand fasting. Besides confusing it with starvation, many believe they cannot survive even a day or two without food. Take, for example, the situation created during the winter of 1978. One weekend in early February, a blizzard that weather forecasters and historians later labeled "the worst storm of the century" hit the northeastern states. Boston, among other cities, was snowed in for a week. But despite the fact that some stores remained open in most places and the fact that most households keep a supply of some extra food on the shelf, a few newspapers carried stories quoting authorities warning that starvation threatened. Of course, no one died during that storm from starvation, although more than twenty died from various other causes. Most persons, even thin ones, have enough body weight to go without food for several days, as long as water is available.

Survival literature relates many stories of stranded adventurers forced to go without food. Mountaineers, Polar explorers, ocean voyagers, airplane crash victims, and others have lived through periods ranging to as many as sixty days without food. (In other cases, humans have turned to cannibalism when the need for food became critical.) Those who sweated it out without food report various horror stories: teeth falling out, wounds not healing, skin color changing, and stomach pain. They became weak, tired, and depressed. Through it all, visions of food permeated every thought. They recalled past family holiday dinners and longed even for liver or brussels sprouts or other foodstuffs they disliked.

But these are involuntary fasts, colored by the knowledge that they cannot be ended when necessary. Life itself is a question mark. Other pain inflicted by the survival situation distorts the feelings of hunger. Fasting advocates vehemently distinguish between starvation and fasting. The very words derive from different roots, they say. Both come from Anglo-Saxon, but starvation came from a word that meant "to die," while fasting descended from a word that meant merely "to go without food" or "to be strict."

Quite simply (we will get to the details later), fasting involves going without food while the body consumes its own stores of extra flesh. Because the body needs protein at all times, some lean muscle tissue as well as fat tissue dissolves during a fast. But, generally, a faster resumes eating before too much lean tissue is lost. As soon as eating begins, the body replaces the lean tissue it poached during the fast. Fasting only becomes starving when the excess flesh the body stores for such emergencies is depleted and the body begins to metabolize essential tissue. When that occurs depends on many factors, including original body weight, body fat content, physical condition, environment, and so on. There are many ground rules fasters must follow to avoid permanent harm to the body, but the main one is this: if, after fasting for several days, hunger returns, stop fasting and begin a period of refeeding. In November 1977, newspapers recounted an incident in Pennsylvania where the rule was tragically violated. A twenty-six-year-old Princeton University graduate, fasting in connection with his practice of yoga, died of starvation. No one knows how long he had fasted, but his weight dropped from at least 145 pounds to at most 80 pounds, doctors estimated.

Another documented and widely quoted death from fasting involves a twenty-year-old English woman who had fasted for thirty weeks, under the care of doctors, to lose weight. Indeed she was successful, shedding almost half her body weight and going from 260 pounds to 132 pounds. She died nine days after she began eating again, two days after her heart started beating irregularly.

Both deaths were needless. If each person had responded to his or her own body signals, the deaths probably would not have occurred. Many fasters have gone on fasting for as long or longer without permanent damage. The champ, according to the *Guinness Book of World Records*, is a man named Angus Barbieri, a Scotsman who took nothing but water, soda water, tea, coffee, and vitamins for 382 days between June 1965 and July 1966. Barbieri's weight declined from 472 pounds to 178 pounds.

Other obese patients have gone on medically supervised fasts for about eight months. One thirty-year-old woman took no food for 236 days, losing 97 pounds before quitting at a weight of 184. A fifty-four-year-old woman stopped eating for 249 days, during which she shed 74 pounds.

But many nonobese and even some thin people fast regularly, for health reasons. They claim it detoxifies their bodies and gives parts of the body a chance to rest. Some swear fasting is therapeutic, letting the body purge itself of diseases as varied as syphilis, cancer, and arthritis. In fact, if you had never heard the word before but listened to some proponents describe it, you'd swear it was a patent medicine, a cure-all. Most of the medical world gives the shortest possible shrift to these claims. Many physicians do not even recognize its use as a weight reducer, even for the very obese. Take a look at the index of a medical textbook sometime—most have no listing under "fasting." Then check for "starvation"; that is where you will find information on fasting.

Many average nonobese persons could survive the Biblical forty-day fast, but even fasting proponents do not suggest undertaking one of that length. At most, you could try fasting for about a month. Twenty days is much safer, and many doctors believe that any fast of ten days or more should be conducted at a hospital. By and large, it is essentially safe to fast by yourself, without medical supervision, only for a day or two, if you follow the rules. Various sources give the record for duration of fasting by a nonobese person to a fakir living in India. In the early 1950s, he went for eighty-one days with nothing but water. But others say that was undocumented. They say the record belongs to Terence MacSwiney, the Irish rebel and mayor of Cork, who went on a hunger strike for seventy-four days before dying of starvation in his British prison cell.

These are only a few of the millions of examples over the centuries that a faster can follow. People in almost every country in the world have a tradition of fasting for some reason. Yet it still seems strange that in the context of today's world, with an increasing interest in food in the United States, more and more Americans tried fasting during the 1960s and 1970s. Why? What made this ancient custom come into vogue again?

On the surface, an old German proverb—"Fasting today makes the food good tomorrow"—would seem to make the most sense. But this time, at least, that wasn't it. We had other reasons to try fasting.

2

why fasting is blossoming

Today fasting may just be a fad. Tomorrow it may be forgotten. In the future, it may be an every-week fact of life, some sages suggest. Fasting seems to be subject to the same human whims as other customs, swinging in and out of fashion with the times. Indeed, in some ways it is. But there is something peculiar about fasting, something unique. Is there another custom that sprang from primitive instincts but endures to this day in essentially unaltered form? True, it now survives for more reasons than those of its original meaning—but that in itself is peculiar. Is there another single phenomenon that has such religious, supernatural, political, and physiological connections? These traditions combine to make fasting more pervasive than is immediately apparent. Although its visible popularity recurs in cycles, there is a certain baseline number of persons for whom going without food every once in a while is simply something one does throughout life, regardless of the public's collective opinion at the moment. If you think about it, you probably know or know of someone like that—that trim little fifty-four-year-old woman down the street who is eating every time you see her, but won't tell you how she diets; the Jewish man who fasts for twenty-four hours a few days each year; the actor or actress or model you just read about who has to stay slim to hold down jobs; the Mexicans who, wanting to become U.S. citizens, employed one of the most effective political pressure techniques by fasting at the front door of the White House two years ago.

Through it all, fasting remains controversial. Ask questions about it and you will hear glowing endorsements. "Fasting changed my life, it changed my whole attitude about food," said one thirtyish Washingtonian who now fasts for several days several times a year. "I feel healthier, trimmer, more independent and more energetic now that it has become part of my routine." Or you will hear vigorous opposition: "I'm against it, for almost every reason. It shouldn't be done for more than a matter of hours. It can be dangerous," says Dr. Robert E. Hodges, the physician who teaches nutrition courses at the University of California at Davis Medical School. Both sides acknowledge that fasting is not as simple as it looks. Anyone who plans to try going without food even for only twenty-four hours should know and abide by certain ground rules that will preclude, at the least, discomfort and, at the most, damage to health.

Nobody knows how many people fast, and no one is likely to learn. Fasting is not the type of subject that would show up in a Gallup or Harris poll. Nor would the U.S. Census Bureau surveys touch on the subject. Picture, if you can, this scene in an ordinary American home.

"Honey, I'm filling out the census. What do you suppose they mean by this—'Have you ever tried fasting?' Have those kids given some new meaning to 'fasting'? They couldn't possibly mean going without food. I mean, a person has to eat."

No, that scene would never happen. Already there are too many important sociological questions left off government surveys because of time, space, and manpower constraints. The government would not take up the question of fasting.

Nor would business, the other grand information collector, underwrite such a survey. Corporations don't want or need the information. There is almost no business associated with fasting—no prospect for profits, no need for data.

There is, in fact, no real value in knowing how many persons throughout the United States or throughout the world do fast. A peculiarly solitary habit, its practice affects almost no one else but the individual doing it. As Ella Wheeler Wilcox once wrote: "Feast, and your halls are crowded; Fast, and the world goes by." The number of people going without food on any one day is minuscule, compared to world population.

Then who cares? Why bother with fasting?

It is interesting because it has survived the ages, growing from its uses in prehistory to many more applications today. It passes as a religious custom, a weight-reducing diet, a way to extend scarce food supplies, a tool of protest for those who cannot exert influence in any other way, a health therapy, and a means to induce supernatural experiences. Fasting transcends various religions, national boundaries, and socioeconomic classes. And while it does not pervade any culture, it is an element of most.

FUTURE FACTS

Fasting is common today and it could conceivably become more common in the future. Although futurologists have not yet predicted that this will happen, several items suggest that it could very easily. Sometime during the last fifty years, Americans began to eat more food than they had previously. This happened gradually and, by 1970, each year each person was consuming (on the average) more than 183 pounds of meat, almost 12 pounds of fish, about 50 pounds of poultry, and 98 pounds of dairy products in addition to 264 pounds of fluid milk and cream, more than 53 pounds of fats and oils, about 81 pounds of fruits, 98 pounds of vegetables, 102 pounds of refined sugar, 110 pounds of wheat flour, and almost 21 pounds of corn sugar and syrup—and those are just the major food commodities listed by the U.S. Department of Commerce in its *Social Indicators 1976* volume of statistics and trends. But this recent pattern of increasing food consumption departs from past trends. Over the years and centuries, as hard physical chores on the job and in the home gave way to technological developments that made men and women more sedentary, people have adjusted by eating less. The health scientists are hoping that this long-term trend resumes and continues. If it does not, Americans face increasing amounts of excess flesh. The prospect makes health care professionals shudder. Obesity may already be the most serious health problem in the United States. Statistics indicate that already at least one-fourth of the adult population is overweight to a degree that threatens health and longevity.

In the past, until the last century, obesity was not much of a medical problem. The medical profession did not have to contend with many degenerative diseases, period. People died at younger ages, before they became feeble.

If Americans continue to eat more, there will be serious problems. Even if they continue to consume about the same amount of food, the dimensions of the associated health problems could escalate. As Dr. George F. Cahill, Jr., of Harvard University told a group of reporters covering the Second International Congress on Obesity held in Weshington, D.C. in 1977: "Obesity is getting worse. But if we go to a three- or four-day workweek, as some have suggested, we ain't seen nothing yet."

Neither Cahill nor his colleagues practicing or researching bariatrics—the medical specialty that treats overweight patients—suggest that fasting is the answer to the obesity problem. But fasting proponents suggest that it could be. In the future, as lives in general become even more sedentary, many may solve their weight maintenance problems by fasting one day a week. Those that already do so indicate it is much easier to go without eating anything for one day, to maintain correct weight, than it is to cut back on caloric intake for several.

The future, in effect, also may make it much easier to fast. "An average of seven thousand new food products are introduced into our markets annually," New York Congressman Frederick Richmond announced at the opening of a series of hearings on nutrition education in the United States. In many cases, manufacturers are substituting cheaper, longer-lasting, or more convenient ingredients for nutritious ones. Because the primary goal of the food industry is efficiency, something less than tasty often results. Giving up fabricated food items that feel like sponge rubber and taste like cardboard can hardly compare in degree of difficulty with passing up a charcoal-broiled T-bone steak, a baked potato with sour cream, and pecan pie a la mode. (Of course, this element would only affect the older generations; young ones brought up on the fabricated items wouldn't be able to recall and savor the good old days when food was real.)

Actually, more serious elements of the future will demand

changes in the nature of food and food consumption. Doomsayers paint a dismal picture of a future world that chronically runs out of many resources, including food supplies in some areas. Although those illustrations probably were sketched with too heavy a hand, the fact remains that most of the world's arable land is already in production. Yet it sometimes strains to feed the current population of four billion. Government researchers say as many as a billion persons may already be underfed. "Each day an estimated 30,000 people starve to death," wrote Norman S. Hoffman, professor of health at Bakersfield College, in his 1977 book, *A New World of Health*. How can the land ever produce enough to feed a population projected to grow to between fifteen and thirty billion over the next two hundred years?

More optimistic forecasters say the answer lies, as always, it seems, in technology. Some oil companies already are experimenting with growing single-cell protein in a medium drawn from petroleum. Scientists at the University of California at Los Angeles are studying the extraction of protein for food from tobacco plant leaves. Other researchers are looking into producing edible protein from cellulose in wood, refuse, and agricultural wastes. Eventually, these proteins presumably would be processed into synthetic analogs of cereal, beef, poultry, and other conventional foods. But even this may not be enough.

To be sure, the press of an increased population will change eating habits. The emphasis will have to be on controlling famine and stopping waste of food. In the past, one tool used to extend food supplies has been periodic fasting. Even today some groups have organized fasts to combat famine. One asks members to fast on the fourteenth day of each month to help relieve world hunger. Fasting is no long-term answer to the food dilemma, but it could, if institutions cooperated, help.

TODAY'S FASTERS

The famine fighters represent only one type of today's faster. You may already be acquainted with several others. If not, listen carefully as you walk down the street—you may hear strollers talking about it. Or ask people you know if they know anyone who fasts. You may be surprised at how often you will run across someone who does. Fasting is experiencing a renaissance today. Whether it is nearing its peak, has hit a far-reaching plateau of popularity, or will soon—despite predictions of future conditions that make it look attractive—roller-coaster down into near-dormancy, no one can tell for sure. What is evident is that over the last ten or fifteen years, the popularity of fasting increased enormously. There were many reasons for it.

Recent years turned out to be ones in which Americans began reexamining personal habits. As economic growth triggered by war-time spending during the 1940s boomed in the 1960s, money in unprecedented amounts percolated down through the various socioeconomic classes (to all but, as government bureaucrats put it, the hard-core unemployed). For the first time, almost everyone had discretionary, surplus income—money not needed to pay the rent or the mortgage or buy groceries or clothes. This was money people could spend on a new Buick with all the extras, a microwave oven, piano lessons, wall-to-wall shag carpeting, a twenty-four-inch color television, and all the other symbols of success that families always have craved. But what happened? All the new toys and gadgets were not enough.

Luxury goods and leisure time to enjoy them did not create contentment after all. So, although they kept on spending, many Americans also turned inward, looking inside themselves for happiness and "meaning." They began to meditate, to practice yoga, and to talk in jargon that said they were "okay." They searched for new avenues to "awareness," instant enlightenment that could be bought at seminars or in books, and ways to develop psychic powers. When this conspicuous consumption and self-overhaul were carried to extremes, it became laughable. New journalist Tom Wolfe dubbed the 1970s "the Me decade." Describing the trend in *New York* magazine, he wrote, "The old alchemical dream was changing base metals into gold. The new alchemical dream is: changing one's personality—remaking, remodeling, elevating, and polishing one's very self . . . and observing, studying, and doting on it. (Me!)" *The Serial*, Cyra McFadden's deliciously satirical book chronicling such excesses among the residents of Marin County, California, drew many chuckles from readers all over the country (even though many of them weren't far behind the trend-setting, consciousness-raised strivers living north of San Francisco).

Yet this lifestyle reevaluation also produced some sound, substantial changes. People grew serious about the quality of the life they were leading. They began to pay more attention to how daily life influenced health and personality. They realized that changing a bad habit could make them feel better. Many stopped, or at least cut back, their cigarette smoking. Even more people began to exercise. In a recent survey Gallup pollsters found that 47 percent of the population claimed to exercise, about double the proportion that made that statement in the early 1960s. Running and jogging spread throughout the country as if it were not the grueling, painful, if exhilarating, activity that it is. In some circles, wielding a tennis racquet became *de rigueur* for both social and physical reasons; between 1970 and 1975 sales of tennis equipment boomed from less than $75 million annually to more than a half billion dollars. Bicycle sales climbed a more gradual path to a higher peak, almost $1 billion by 1976.

Even more important, people revamped their eating habits. Actually, this is not surprising. Doctors have found that most people, especially those with excess weight, would rather forego that second piece of buttered toast at breakfast, or some such morsel, than walk instead of drive the eight blocks or so to the shopping center. "People are more resistant to increasing exercise than to reducing caloric intake, even in my experiences with behavior modification," confirms Dr. Henry A. Jordan of the University of Pennsylvania. Jordan, a leader in the bariatric school that believes that lifestyle changes are necessary to keep a slimmed-down person from regaining lost weight, is the author of *Eating Is Okay*.

Although the connection between diet and disease remains controversial, evidence implicating certain foods and eating habits as a factor contributing to some diseases has been stacking up in researchers' offices. "Six out of ten of the leading causes of death in this country have been linked to the way we eat," Representative Fred Richmond said in 1977. "Our diet, overrich in fat, cholesterol, refined sugars and starches, salt and alcohol, is associated with epidemic rates of heart disease, cancer, high blood pressure, stroke, hardening of the arteries and cirrhosis." When the news spread that both heart disease, the nation's number one cause of death, and atherosclerosis were related to intake of cholesterol, a waxy fat substance, millions switched from butter to margarine, a less-saturated fat. Consumption of eggs, another cholesterol villain, dropped 26 percent from 1950 to 1974. The average American's cholesterol level has dropped 5 to 10 percent since the early 1960s, the National Heart, Lung and Blood Institute announced in July 1977. And deaths from cardiovascular disease decreased by 15 percent in about the same period. (The facts could not, however, persuade Americans to give up their preference for beef and other high-fat meats. But doctors surmise that most people are buying leaner cuts and are probably being more attentive to trimming fat before they eat meat.)

How does fasting fit in with all of this? Since Americans were now displaying a greater concern for their health and more interest in what they were eating, they had created a climate in which fasting could flourish. Most directly, fasting established a role as a weight-reducer and weight-controller. Doctors believe that excess weight of as little as 20 percent above optimum body weight can impair health. And, in 1977, "at least one-fourth of all adults in the United States are overweight to a degree that jeopardizes health and longevity," Representative Richmond announced. So millions tried fasting as a diet for the first time. Fasting had been used therapeutically to treat obesity since Hippocrates lived more than 2,000 years ago. But modern medical doctors had not really begun experimenting with prolonged fasting as a diet until the late 1950s. By November 1962, word that doctors were prescribing fasting for the very obese had spread to mainstream America. That month *Reader's Digest* printed "A Sure, Swift Way to Take Off Weight," describing the experiences of Dr. Garfield G. Duncan of the University of Pennsylvania School of Medicine. Five months later, *Newsweek* printed a similar story. By late in the decade the not-so-overweight had it taken it up.

Second, somewhere along the way Americans became aware of how bad for health some things found in their diets were. The average American's normal intake of food, for example, now contains more than five pounds of chemical additives, colorings, and preservatives each year. In a touching moment less than a year before he died, Senator Hubert Humphrey reportedly noted at a nutrition hearing that he wished he and the country had developed more information on the connection between nutrition and disease, particularly the roles of additives, long ago. It may have, he said, prevented his own problem, bladder cancer, and countless others like it. Many fasters have heeded that warning. They already avoid additive-tainted food whenever possible. But doing that precludes the use of any canned or processed food—these days, almost an impossibility. So they fast for a day or two every so often to cleanse the body from the chemicals that may have been building up.

Third, many people became interested in offbeat medical cures. Many began to doubt the infallibility of technology. Sales of vitamins thrived as it became known that some scientists, many with good credentials, such as Nobel prizewinner Linus Pauling, believed that large doses of vitamin C could cure the common cold. Other vitamins could in other ways improve health or counteract disease, some claimed. Health food stores featuring vitamins and various dietary supplements sprang up all over the country, even in small towns. A small magazine named *Prevention*, first published in 1950, touted "healthful" living practices—sometimes of dubious value—to prevent disease. By early 1978, the magazine's circulation had climbed to almost 1.2 million. In this context, it was only natural for fasting to again show its head as a way both to prevent and to cure illness. The idea is not new; advocates claim to draw their inspiration from animals, who supposedly stop eating when sick. Practitioners can trace therapeutic fasting back at least a hundred years in the United States.

The new emphasis on health also boosted the practice of yoga, and to a yogi (one who practices yoga) fasting is an integral part of the purification process he or she goes through.

The yoga boom brings up another important trend of the last several years that helped to foster fasting—the renewal of interest in Eastern religions. Both Hinduism and Buddhism encourage yoga as a spiritual exercise. Other religions, too, went through and are still going through revivals. Although today fasting is not as important as a religious ritual as it was centuries ago, it is still a part of most religions in either personal or group practice.

One last trend of the 1960s and 1970s contributed to fasting's renaissance: the protest movement. The Vietnam war politicized many middle Americans. Many who had in the past remained silent on the issues of the day began to sense the illegitimacy of the war. Those more staunch in their opposition turned to more dramatic gestures of protest. Along with the bombings, the rallies, the marches, and the sit-ins, there was mass and personal fasting. In other parts of the world—Ireland, Africa, England, and Germany come to mind—there were other actions to protest. Many who did took up the weapon of fasting.

In short, fasting became popular again because its principle connections did. Religion, political protest, dieting, and health each experienced a revival. And fasting has been entwined with each since they began.

3
origin and folklore

"Now why didn't I think of that?"

You've heard people say that hundreds of times. With the subject of fasting, the sentiment is usually the other way around: many people question why anyone would invent anything as disagreeable as voluntary fasting. Recognizing the unpleasantness involved, most people believe that fasting originated as a religious practice of penance. They are wrong. Organized religions are only a few thousand years old, and fasting goes back much further than that.

If we really knew how old the earth and the various forms of life that it supports are, we might be able to date fasting. But we can only speculate. The exact origin of fasting is lost, yet anthropologists believe its practice among human beings goes back to the very beginning of society. It was probably born of necessity. In the earliest cultures, man depended solely on his environment to satisfy his needs. These men and women gathered their food from the wilds. Later they took up hunting and fishing. But there was no system—they sought food when they were hungry, often gorging, eating all they found immediately. When food was scarce, they had no alternative except "fasting," involuntary though it may have been. Eventually, they put a little organization into their subsistence, storing food for later use. Short, intermittent fasts became a way of extending existing food reserves when supplies looked tight. Primitive peoples may have borrowed this idea of fasting from animals, who supposedly do it instinctively. Some animals in cold or temperate areas hibernate during winter scarcity, taking no food and going into a dormant state. In more tropical climates, some animals similarly reduce their food consumption and activity level during hot or dry months; they aestivate.

Of course, this measure for avoiding hunger did not prove to be enough. So man learned to plant and harvest foodstuffs. Some anthropologists think agricultural economies, too, used the fasting trick when famine threatened. If the rains were late in coming or thin in volume, these early societies easily could have recognized that they should begin to conserve their food stores. So they spread out what food they had as long as possible. Sometimes they could have had to resort to short periods of fasting. Complete abstention from food, a few days at a time now and then, is usually easier than eating sparingly throughout the same period.

If fasting started purely as a practical response to environmental conditions, however, it probably did not remain so limited very long. Man also has a craving for magic and mystery, a need that is especially high in primitive cultures. Perhaps because of the euphoria fasting is said to excite, its practice became bound up with magic and ritual. As fasting spread, it picked up many meanings. Even among the primitive societies that exist today, anthropologists have discovered fasting rituals.

The first step to concluding that fasting has magical power was easy. Lacking any better reason, early men and women thought that they became sick because they ate certain foods. Sometimes they thought a particular piece of food itself was the villain that caused the disease. But they also believed in ghosts and spirits and, on other occasions, they thought that the food was inhabited by a demon that was doing the harm. When they became sick, they stopped eating, either avoiding the one kind of food or abstaining altogether. It usually worked; they got well, although it was probably the body curing itself. Man deduced that fasting—miraculously, it seemed to him—could cure disease. And if the disease had been brought on by a demon, then fasting could drive evil spirits away. If fasting worked on illness-causing evil spirits, it could probably repel other demons, too.

To some extent, this belief survives even in today's civilized societies. In a celebrated case that took place in West Germany in 1976, fasting reportedly played a part in the exorcism of a twenty-three-year-old woman. The eleven-month rites ended in her death from malnutrition and dehydration. A year later, in the United States, Indianapolis police discovered a six-year-old boy dead from malnutrition and dehydration. They found five other children in only slightly better condition. One relative told authorities that the six had been fed only salt water for several days as part of a rite to drive away demons.

Fasting, then, evolved into a purification ceremony. When a crime was committed, for example, fasting could wash away the taint and the guilt. In the western mountains of Ecuador, where the Jibaro Indians lived, a purification ceremony could even absolve one of murder. When a man killed his enemy, he was painted with blood and made to dance. A period of fasting followed. His wife had to undergo the same rite. The fasting signifies seeking of pardon; the blood is a symbol of the dead person's soul. The ceremony protects the murderer from the revenge of his spirit. In some cultures, fasting also purified a person in the sense of making him worthy of something that was about to happen. Among the Chibcha Indians of Colombia, the heir to the throne was made to endure a long probation. The Chibchas claim to be the original children of the Sun, their deity, and they lavished their monarch with gold, other riches, and unlimited powers. But in preparation for becoming monarch, the heir had to give up worldly pleasures for at least five years. He lived in seclusion in a temple, where he fasted for long periods. Between fasts, he was whipped and subjected to other humiliations.

North American Indians in the area bordering the north shores of the Gulf of Mexico held an annual purification ceremony in July or August. These were the Muskhogean Indians, including the Creeks, Choctaws, Chickasaws, Seminoles, Alabamas, and Apalachees. White people called the ceremony "the Busk," a corruption of a Creek word "*puskita*," which means the fast. The Busk was celebrated whenever the maize first matured, but it was more like a New Year's celebration and carried all the connotations of renewal and rejuvenation of all life. For eight days (sometimes four days in smaller towns and villages), everyone fasted and refrained from sex. The town was cleaned; old pots, vessels, and mats were destroyed. Fires were put out. Then new vessels were made, new medicines were brewed, and a new fire was kindled from friction. The Indians bathed in running water, prepared a sacrifice of the first fruits of the harvest, and began a new hunt. All crimes except murder were forgiven. There were dances and, in the end, there was a grand feast.

The Busk illustrates the common practice of fasting before a harvest, or a hunt, to separate new food from old food. Many cultures believed the two should not be mixed; the fast purifies the body in the interval.

Once primitive cultures attributed to fasting the powers of purification and expulsion of demons, people started believing it had other magical powers. Some used it as a weapon or a tool to make what they desired happen. Celtic folklore, for example, includes the story of a mythical Saint Finnen. His enemy, a great warrior, is hiding inside an unbreachable fortress. But Finnen succeeds at getting inside by fasting against his enemy.

In another Celtic myth, three saints and several poets lament the loss of the Táin, a beautiful, long narrative poem that had not been recorded. A dead man named Fergus can recite the poem (whether he wrote it is unclear), so Saints Brendan, Columba, and Ciaran, as well as the poets, fast at the grave of Fergus, making him appear and saving the poem from oblivion.

Fasting has long been thought to make communing with the dead possible, an idea that later turns up in a slightly different form among the Hebrews. One explanation suggests that giving up food eliminates one distinction between the living and the dead and makes communication easier. Another says fasting allows a living person's soul to separate from the body, permitting it to travel to the world of the dead. Some historians disagree, however; they say fasting was the way of providing nourishment for the dead, perhaps during a transitory state between this world and the next. In any case, fasting became common during periods of mourning and thereafter, when someone wanted to talk with the dead.

In another twist, fasting was used to fend off death. If it could cure disease, why couldn't it prevent illness and prolong life? Many cultures, even more sophisticated ones, thought that it could. In ancient China, for example, historians have discovered literature that describes fasting, called *p'i ku*, as the most important of the "cordials of immortality."[1]

Most American Indian tribes believed that their medicine men drew their powers to cure from a past-induced vision. Medicine men would teach a candidate for their trade the procedures and principles and ceremonies, but then the neophyte had to go off to the wilderness on his first *hanblechia* (vision quest), as the Sioux called it. Listen to John Fire Lame Deer tell his story, as he wrote it in *Lame Deer—Seeker of Visions*.

> *I was all alone on the hilltop. I sat there in my vision pit, a hole dug into the hill, my arms hugging my knees as I watched old man Chest, the medicine man who had brought me there, disappear down into the valley. . . . Now I was all by myself, left on the hilltop for four days and nights without food or water until he came back for me . . . left alone by myself for the first time in my life.*

Later, as he huddles with a special quilt his grandmother had made for the occasion and with a peace pipe and red bark tobacco, the vision comes.

> *Suddenly I felt an overwhelming presence. . . . I was no longer myself . . . slowly I perceived that a voice was trying to tell me something. It was a bird cry, but I can tell you, I began to understand some of it. . . . I heard a human voice too, strange and high-pitched, a voice which could not come from an ordinary, living being.*

The four days had passed, the old medicine man Chest came up to get Lame Deer, and he became a medicine man for the Sioux.

Although Lame Deer had been specially trained and was fasting to receive his medicine-man powers, he was also undergoing a rite of passage into manhood. Almost without exception, American Indian tribes prescribed a period of fasting at puberty as an initiation rite. Most primitive societies put their boys through

[1] Louis Herbert Gray, ed., *The Mythology of All Races* (New York: Cooper Square Publishers, 1964), Vol. 8, p. 146.

various physical ordeals to prove their masculinity. Fasting demonstrates control of the body and therefore strength, an adequate test of manhood.

Enduring this trial usually conveyed various rewards—a new, adult name, the right to kill, the right to own a horse, sometimes even the right to choose a mate or to have sexual intercourse. Among some tribes, such as the Ojibways of Minnesota and Wisconsin, passing the test of a long fast promised a long life of comfort and plenty. The Ojibways, part of the Algonquin nation, also required women to endure the fasting ordeal at puberty, as did some other tribes.

There was good reason for this. The Ojibways were seeking communion with a spirit that would guard and guide them throughout life. They were a deeply religious people, and they did not dare to communicate directly with the "One Great Master of Life," to whom all other spirits were subordinate. Their personal guardian spirit, sometimes called a totem, acted as a mediator for them with the supreme being.

The rite of fasting took on this religious meaning in most Indian tribes. Fasting purified the body, already a factor in other Indian traditions. It made the adolescent fit to acquire his personal guardian spirit. Since the fasting occurred in the wilderness, the youth was isolated from the rest of society, allowing him to purify his mind, too, as he contemplated the coming experience. When the mind and body were both purified (most tribes did not have a specific, required length of time for this), the spirit would come in a vision or a dream. The spirit would often take on the form of an ordinary object or animal—a moose, an elk, a rock, a butterfly, the tail of a snake. It would bring knowledge and guidance, and it was expected to warn its ward of danger throughout life. Then it would disappear. An Indian could appeal to his guardian for help or direction in times of emergency. At various times throughout life, an Indian would go back into the wilderness to fast and to pray, hoping that a revelation from his guardian would help him out of some difficulty. Sometimes secret societies were formed among those who had the same guardian spirit. They often played a major part in an Indian's life.

But, except for knowing these things and knowing that the intimate relationship between an Indian and his spirit continued throughout life, we know little else about what happened during the fasting, the sacred rite of passage. Paul Radin writes in *The Story of the American Indian*: "The blessings vouchsafed by the spirits to a youth during his adolescent fasting was too holy, too personal a thing ever to be divulged. It meant life."

This cult of the guardian spirit is distinctly North American, but the idea of fasting as an initiation, a purification, a way of seeking guidance or expelling demons, and in its other constituent elements is common elsewhere in primitive religions. And when the time came for worship of a supreme being or for many gods to be organized into identifiable religions, fasting was not forgotten.

4

religious traditions

FROM A MOUNTAINTOP in the old city of Kabul, Afghanistan's capital, a cannon erupts in the still, predawn hours, announcing the beginning of the holiest month in the Islamic year. At the same time, another cannon blast imparts the same message in Cairo. In Muslim villages, shotguns fire. Elsewhere, Muslim priests climb to the minarets of their mosques to proclaim that the new moon has been seen in Mecca.

It is Ramadan. For the next thirty days, until religious elders sight the next new moon, the entire nation of Islam fasts according to rules set down by the Prophet Muhammad. From daybreak until sundown, they take no food or drink. After dark, they should eat sparingly, although today many do not. And at the end of Ramadan they celebrate *Eid ul Fitr*, the "Festival of the Breaking of the Fast." It is the year's most joyous holiday, a Christmas and New Year's rolled into one celebration.

At about the same time of year in 1977, Jews throughout the world were observing Yom Kippur, the most solemn day on the Jewish calendar. On this Day of Atonement Jews take no food or drink, not even water, for twenty-four hours, "from even to even." As the only fast prescribed by Mosaic law, most Jews keep Yom Kippur strictly. God ordered the fast when he spoke to Moses in the third book of the Bible, Leviticus (16:29–31): "On the tenth day of the seventh month you shall mortify yourselves; you shall do no work, whether native Israelite or alien settler, because on this day expiation shall be made on your behalf to cleanse you, and so make you clean before the Lord from all your sins. This is a sabbath of sacred rest for you, and you shall mortify yourselves; it is a rule binding for all time." (In this and other passages of the Bible, the words "mortify yourself" can be translated to mean "fast." Literally, the Hebrew word *tzwm* means abstinence from food, but the Hebrews also used an idiom, *innah nefesh*, which literally means "afflict the body," to mean "fast." In most translations of the Bible, however, *innah nefesh* is translated either literally or as "mortify yourself.")

So ordered by God, the world's fifteen million Jews stay home from work, fast, and worship at the temple on Yom Kippur.

Despite the differences in these two and other specific customs, the practice of fasting runs as a common thread through the fabric of most organized faiths. It is most tightly woven into the ritual of Islam and Judaism, but Catholics, Hindus, Buddhists, Mormons, Eastern Orthodox, Anglicans, and most other faiths have some fasting tradition—sometimes public, sometimes private, sometimes formal and prescribed, sometimes unwritten custom. Organized religions grew out of the same instinctive needs that earlier cultures fulfilled with their mythologies—the search for an understanding of life, the universe, the future, and a personal relationship with the Supreme Being. Fasting was instinctively a part of this. Sometimes it was an attempt to imitate the gods. People living on Nias, an island off the western coast of Sumatra, include fasting in their creation myth; they believe that the Supreme Being fasted for many days after the creation of the world, whereas most traditional creation stories only suggest that God rested. Other cultures thought God or the gods had no need for food. Most frequently, fasting serves as a penance, a means of gaining God's favors, and a purification ceremony. Many religions also follow a tradition of "fast before feast." Almost all claim that fasting brings a spiritual joy.

The ancients generally observed fasting rules and traditions far more faithfully than today's believers do. Now the practice ranges widely, from Roman Catholicism, for example, where a once strong tradition has eroded to the point of almost no organized observance, to Islam, where fasting, albeit often in the diluted form already described, remains a fundamental tenet.

ISLAMIC FASTS

For a Muslim, keeping the Ramadan fast is like going to a Christmas Day or Easter service for a Christian. It is one of the rules that must be kept, even if other religious practices have been abandoned. It fulfills the letter of the law, at least, if the spirit is lacking. Ramadan fasting is an absolute requirement of Islam, the fourth of the Five Pillars. (The other four obligatory duties are reciting a profession of faith, praying, paying a tax to the mosque, and making a pilgrimage to Mecca.)

It was during Ramadan, the ninth month of the Islamic year and literally "the scorcher," that the contents of the Koran were revealed to Muhammad. And the Koran, guide to the will of Allah, who is God, specifically enjoins the Ramadan fast: "Until you can distinguish a white thread from a black thread in the dawn; then keep the fast until night; do not mix with women, but retire to places of worship" (Koran, sura ii, v. 183). All physically able adult Muslims are supposed to fast during Ramadan; the sick, those traveling, women near childbirth, and a few others may seek dispensations. They must later make up the days missed. The command is taken very seriously; some Muslim countries used to compel those reluctant to fast by locking them up.

In these predominantly Muslim areas, the beginning of Ramadan is announced ceremonially, if not by gunshot then by lighting of lamps. On each day following, the faster gets up before dawn to make a *niya*, an intention, for that day. Alternately, a Muslim can decide on an intention for the entire month.

The fast is meant to atone for transgressions against Allah's will, and devout Muslims keep the difficult rules of the Ramadan fast very strictly. They abide by a rule that says that nothing—not a pin, a toothbrush, a pencil, or any instrument—may enter any part of the body during daylight hours. Food, drink, and sexual intercourse, of course, are explicitly forbidden. Even spittle is not supposed to be swallowed. One may not inhale tobacco smoke. Because the days are holy days, Muslims are supposed to avoid anything that gives sensual pleasure or arouses passion. They should also make special efforts to refrain from minor wrongs such as lying or giving insults.

Things let up after sunset. The faster thanks Allah, then takes a little food. Recalling the Bedouin culture in which Islam took root, tradition dictates that the faster break the fast by eating ripe dates. Very strict Muslims with a Bedouin heritage still follow that recommendation. Others may let a date be the first morsel to cross their lips, but then they move on to heartier fare. Still others follow newer traditions. In Egypt, for example, a Muslim usually breaks the fast with a dish of a national specialty, brown beans cooked with lemon, oil, and spices, or a bowl of soup. Later, during the night, the faster can take another meal, preferably right before dawn.

Even though the meals during Ramadan were never supposed to be banquets, many Muslims today admit that they eat more during that month than they do during other months. This is especially true when Ramadan falls during the summer (the Muslim calendar is set by the lunar calendar, and thus the months move around within the Western calendar in a rotating cycle), because hot weather makes fasting—especially without water—more difficult. Many countries find it prudent to shorten the workday during Ramadan, not necessarily because the Muslims have not eaten enough to sustain themselves during full working hours, but because many of them stay up much of the night eating. (Muslim rules, by the way, denounce sleeping during the day to avoid the hunger pangs and thirst of the fast.)

The rules are not so strict, however, that they do not leave room for mistakes. Actual slipups are forgiven; breaking the fast must be deliberate. "If one eats by oversight," says the Islamic Traditions, "he may continue the fast because God himself caused him to eat."

The promised rewards of keeping the fast are great. As Muhammad himself proclaimed in the Traditions, "There are two pleasures in fasting, one when the person who fasts breaks it, and the other in the next world when he meets his Lord. The very smell of the mouth of a keeper of a fast is more agreeable to God than the smell of musk."

Still, while devout Muslims observe the Ramadan fast very carefully, the unity in which whole Muslim countries kept the fast is no longer. The tradition remains strong in the Arab world; elsewhere it is gradually falling off, particularly among the young, who are no longer as religious as their parents and grandparents. In some places, even though fasting is not required until one reaches puberty, young children used to try to fast for the first day or two of Ramadan in an attempt to be grown up. Proud grandparents would make a fuss over how good the children were. But there is less and less of such enthusiasm.

Muslims fast as penance for their sins, just as members of most religions do. Since Ramadan was unlikely to make up for an entire year's transgressions, Muhammad set aside other days for fasting. He selected the tenth day of Muharram, and called it the Ashura Day, as a day to prepay for sins in the coming year. Immediately after the Festival of the Breaking of the Fast, he chose another period, saying in the Traditions, "The person who fasts the month of Ramadan, and follows it up with six days of the month of Shawwal, will obtain the rewards of a continued fast."

Muhammad suggested that devout Muslims fast on Monday and Thursday of every week, the days on which he said God pays particular attention to the actions of humans, and the thirteenth, fourteenth, and fifteenth of every month. He also prescribed, through the Koran, fasting as penance for specific transgressions—slightly out-of-date today. Killing game while on a pilgrimage, for example, merits two months of fasting, as does killing a believer of an allied nation by accident. Some could still hold, however, such as a three-day fast to make up for breaking an oath. Although Muhammad observed these days and these rules himself, not all of today's 500 million Muslims follow his example. Some have never even heard of the more obscure rules.

These personal fasts, however, are held in the highest esteem among the religious because, theoretically, only God and not others see the acts of self-denial. "Every good act that a man does shall receive from ten to seven hundred rewards, but the rewards of fasting are beyond bounds, for fasting is for God alone, and he will give its rewards," Muhammad says in the Traditions.

Second, Islamic belief states that fasting can help one to avoid sin. Muslims think, and many modern individuals would agree, that eating and drinking arouses human desires or at least intensifies them, often leading the faithful to stray.

Though Ramadan fasting later became one of Islam's Five Pillars, Muhammad did not prescribe it when he first began preaching his new religion in Mecca, now part of Saudi Arabia. The time was the early part of the seventh century, and Mecca's inhabitants worshiped animistic spirits and idols. Muhammad attracted some followers, but he also incurred hostility from others. When he learned of a plot to assassinate him, he fled to Medina. There he met Christians and Jews and learned of their custom of fasting. At first, he patterned the Ashura Day after Yom Kippur, making it a one-day mandatory fast. Later he changed his mind, made Ashura a voluntary fast, and instituted the month-long Ramadan tradition.

JEWISH FASTS

The Jews Muhammad saw, of course, were steeped in knowledge of the Bible, and they drew their inspiration to fast from it. Jewish authorities agree that Jews began fasting very early in history, probably before some parts of the Bible were written. The custom was not in the least unusual in the Near Eastern culture of the times. Historical accounts of the seagoing Phoenicians, who invented the modern alphabet around 1000 B.C., tell about fasting. These famed traders lived in what is today Syria and Lebanon, but they traveled around the entire Mediterranean region. They transmitted many customs from one culture to another, and fasting may have been one of them.

The Bible relates many instances of fasting; some editions mention it on at least seventy-five occasions. For inspiration, the Jews need look no further than Moses. Moses, in fact, is the Bible's first faster. His story is told in Exodus, the second look of the Bible. The time is the thirteenth century B.C. Moses is leading the Jews out of Egypt through the desert to the Promised Land. He climbs Mount Sinai to make a covenant with God. But before he descends with the Ten Commandments, "Moses stayed there with the Lord forty days and forty nights, neither eating nor drinking, and wrote down the words of the covenant, the Ten Words, on the tablet" (Exodus 34:28).

With so many examples to follow, fasting soon became an integral part of Judaism. One whole tractate of the Talmud, the *Megillat Ta'amit*, which translates as "The Scroll of Fasting," concentrates on the practice. It lists about twenty-five days on which it recommends that Jews fast. Each day commemorates a Biblical or historical event. The book of Esther, for example, relates a suspenseful tale that is today celebrated in the feast of Purim. It tells of King Ahasueris who, unknowingly married to a Jewess, the beautiful orphan Esther, consents to a plot advanced by his evil assistant to murder all Jews in his Kingdom. At first, Esther keeps her secret, fearing for her own life and also afraid to violate a tradition that mandates death for those who enter the Persian king's presence unsummoned. But her foster father Mordecai pressures her, preying on her conscience and warning that she might not escape the massacre. Finally, she agrees to intervene for her people, saying, "Go and assemble all the Jews to be found in Susa and fast for me; take neither food nor drink for three days, night or day, and I and my maids will fast as you do. After that I will go to the king, although it is against the law; and if I perish, I perish" (Esther 4:16). Mordecai organizes the community fast, Esther intercedes with the king, and the Jews are spared. Today, Jews mark the eve of Purim, which is the thirteenth of Adar on the Hebrew calendar, with a fast. The next day is celebrated as one of the most festive holy days of the year, symbolizing religious freedom.

True to the troubled history of the Jews, most of their fast days commemorate tragic events. Several recall the deaths of important leaders, such as Miriam the prophetess, the high priests Aaron and Eli, the prophet Samuel, and Joshua and Moses. Others remind Jews of the assassination of Gedaliah, governor of Judah, the breaching of Jerusalem's walls in the sixth century B.C., and the siege of Jerusalem by Babylonian King Nebuchadnezzar.

A community's elders held the power to proclaim a public fast, generally when they sensed a disaster coming. By fasting they asked God to help them escape it. These fasts usually lasted one day or three days, sometimes as many as seven days. Some emergency fasts, like Esther's, later became permanent fast days on the calendar. As another Biblical story unfolds, for example, some Israelites are fighting an internecine war against the Benjaminites. Twice defeated on the battlefields, they retreat to mourn their dead and to plot new strategy. The elders declare a public fast (Judges 20:26) and offer sacrifice to God. Back at war, they trounce the Benjaminites. In honor of this victory, the *Megillat Ta'amit* suggests a fast on the twenty-third day of the month of Shebat. These mandated fasts also worked in other emergencies—ending a famine caused by a plague of locusts, winning forgiveness for community misdeeds, and helping Israel defeat the Philistines and its Transjordanian enemies.

Private fasts became common, too. Individuals, particularly women, often went without food once or twice a week, either to strengthen their will to avoid sin or in reparation for sins committed. "Fasting is more effective than charity," the Talmud says, "for the latter is done with money, but the former can be done only by one's own person."

As people fasted, they believed they became closer to God and more godlike. So, like primitive peoples before them, Hebrews traditionally fasted as preparation for communicating with God, often before they sought and received a divine revelation. Daniel's story is typical; he fasted before he experienced a vision in which the future of the Israelites was revealed to him. "In those days I, Daniel, mourned for three whole weeks. I refrained from all choice food; no meat or wine passed my lips, and I did not anoint myself until three weeks had gone by. . . . I looked up and saw a man clothed in linen with a belt of gold from Ophir round his waist. . . . I, Daniel, alone saw the vision. . . . When he addressed me, I stood up trembling and he said, 'Do not be afraid, Daniel, for from the very first day that you applied your mind to understand and to mortify yourself before your God, your prayers have been heard, and I have come in answer to them' " (Daniel 10:2,3,5,7,12).

In a little-known part of one of the most well-known Bible stories, King David fasted to try to save the life of the son he had fathered by Bathsheba, who was another man's wife. Her husband, Uriah, was fighting in David's army at the time. When Bathsheba became pregnant, David arranged for Uriah to be put on the front lines, where he was killed in battle. Then he took Bathsheba as his wife. But God showed his disapproval by making the boy ill. As the Bible says, "David prayed to God for the child; he fasted and went in and spent the night fasting, lying on the ground. The older men of the household tried to get him to rise from the ground, but he refused and would eat no food with them. On the seventh day the boy died" (II Samuel 12:16–18).

Later, a defiant David violated the custom of fasting when a loved one dies. "Then he went home, asked for food to be brought, and when it was ready, he ate it. His servants asked him, 'What is this? While the boy lived you fasted and wept for him, but now that he is dead you rise up and eat.' He answered, 'While the boy was still alive I fasted and wept thinking, "It may be that the Lord will be gracious to me, and the boy may live." But now that he is dead, why should I fast? Can I bring him back again? I shall go to him; he will not come back to me.' "

Nevertheless, most Jews fasted on private occasions—a death, the anniversary of a parent's death, their wedding day, and others. Private fasting came in and out of fashion over the years. At some points, it became so popular that rabbis began to condemn those who carried it to extremes. They feared some people would become community burdens. Instead, the rabbis told their congregations to avoid sin, so that it would be unnecessary to atone for them in so many fasts. The *Megillat Ta'amit* lists about thirty-five days, joyful events on the Jewish calendar, on which fasting is prohibited.

At other times many tired of fasting, even on fixed fast days. Why is it necessary, they asked on one occasion in the Bible. True, the days commemorated sad events, ending with the destruction of the holy temple in Jerusalem but, for a second time, the Jews had sacrificed to rebuild the temple. Now it stood in its majesty in the old city. In the book of Zechariah, a Jew named Bethel-sharezer sends his men "to seek the favor of the Lord. They were to say to the priests in the house of the Lord of Hosts and to the prophets, 'Am I to lament and abstain in the fifth month as I have done for so many years?' Then the word of the Lord of Hosts came to me: Say to all the people of the land and to the priests, When you fasted and lamented in the fifth and seventh months these seventy years, was it indeed in my honour that you fasted? And when you ate and drank, was it not to please yourselves? Was it not this that the Lord proclaimed through the propets of old, while Jerusalem was populous and peaceful, as were cities round her, and the Negeb and the Shepheleh?" (Zechariah 7:2–7). He continues, "The word of the Lord of Hosts came to me: These are the words of the Lord of Hosts: The fasts of the fourth month and of the fifth, the seventh, and the tenth, shall become festivals of joy and gladness for the house of Judah. Love truth and peace" (Zechariah 8:18–19).

The prophet Isaiah dwelled on fasting in his "warnings to keep the moral law." He railed against impious fasts, calling instead for fasts that embody and accompany acts of charity. "Then shall your light break forth like the dawn and soon you will grow healthy like a wound newly healed; your righteousness shall be your vanguard and the glory of the Lord your rearguard" (Isaiah 58:8).

Today, the two most widely observed fasts among Jews are Yom Kippur, the Day of Atonement, which is kept by all Jews, and the ninth of Av, commemorating the destruction of the two temples in Jerusalem (which Orthodox and Conservative Jews keep, although many reform Jews do not). They abstain from food, drink (even water), and pleasures of any kind. That was the idea behind *innah nefesh* (self-mortification). Fasting only played the lead role in a day of total self-denial. In the old days, that meant wearing sackcloth (and perhaps ashes), abstaining from sex, sleeping on the hard ground instead of in a bed, going barefoot, taking part in a special liturgical worship, and so worth. The rules encouraged Jews to give alms to the poor on these days. But these rules, decreeing a regimen of total self-denial, applied only on the very important fast days, such as Yom Kippur. Ordinary fast days called only for abstinence from food and drink. The important fast days lasted twenty-four hours, while lesser fast days by custom were endured only from sunrise until the first star could be seen in the sky.

Laws of fasting such as these have not changed in essence since Biblical times. The idea of fixed annual fasts first comes up in the Bible in the book of Zechariah, written before Jesus Christ was born, but since then a wealth of information about fasting and Judaism has been written. One rabbi, asked about Jewish fasting customs, threw up his hands in despair. "I can't possibly tell you about it. There is so much to say. I don't even know where to begin—any precept that was set down in the Bible is very carefully explored and developed in later rabbinic literature." Indeed, there are too many customs to put down here. Yet a few more deserve mention. At some times in some places, small children and even domesticated animals were required to fast. First-born males are supposed to fast on the eve of Passover, marking the time first-born sons were spared from death during the tenth plague in Egypt (Exodus 13). If a Torah scroll (the scripture documents used in liturgical services) is dropped, those present must fast. Rabbis often forbade scholars and teachers from fasting, not wanting their strength and diligence for studying the scriptures to be sapped.

Except for observance by very devout Jews, however, most of these customs go unheeded today. There is even some good-humored, but not irreverent, joking about the custom. "It's good to fast—with a chicken leg and a bottle of wine," writes Leo Rosten in his *Treasury of Jewish Quotations*. Fasting seems to be one of the religious practices that has currently gone out of style in the Jewish community. After World War II, Jewish authorities tried to rekindle an interest in the fast days by attaching modern meanings to them. For example, Jews used to fast on the tenth day of the month of Tevet to commemorate the siege of Jerusalem by Babylonian King Nebuchadnezzar; rabbis suggested that the day now memorialize the Jews who perished in the Nazi persecutions. But it has not as yet worked. Except for the one or two days kept by the Jewish community as a whole, fasting remains very much an individual practice among today's Jews.

CHRISTIAN FASTS

Fasting has seen more ups and downs among Christians than among the faithful of any other major religion. At times, a majority of Christians did follow fasting ritual; at other times, there has been no organized observance. If there is one basic reason for this, it is probably that Jesus Christ neither wrote nor prescribed any laws about fasting. He left the subject open to whatever decision his disciples made, and they essentially passed the responsibility on to local churches. Eventually, the Pope ruled on fasting for Roman Catholics. But, by then, Christianity had divided into many different churches, each with its own ritual and customs.

By the time Jesus was spreading his gospel among his fellow Jews in and around Jerusalem, fasting was firmly entrenched in Judaic custom. Jesus himself went out into the desert to fast after his baptism. Following the examples of Moses and the prophet Elijah, he took no food for 40 days as a preparation for beginning his ministry. It was at the end of this fast, after he had been tempted by the devil, that Christ spoke his famous words: "Man cannot live by bread alone; he lives on every word that God utters" (Matthew 4:4).

But when Jesus observed the prevailing religious customs, he was disgusted by the attitudes of the Pharisees, an elite group of supposedly pious scholars who followed a century-old practice of fasting two days a week. The Pharisees prayed many times a day as well, but they also sought praise and recognition of their godliness among men, so much so that it, instead of worshiping God, became their prime goal. Sometimes they even made themselves look gray and ashen so that others would know that they were fasting. Seeing this, Jesus railed against fasting without repentance, noting that fasting is not an end in itself, but a means for man to do penance for sins and to please God. Be humble in all religious practices, he said; be not like the Pharisees.

In this, Christ was simply reiterating what the prophet Isaiah had said before him. Isaiah criticized those who fasted to the letter of the law, but not in the spirit required to make it a religious experience. Much later, Italian Catholics said the same thing in their own irreverent way. One of their proverbs states: "Who fasts but does no other good saves his bread but goes to Hell."

So although Christ did not repudiate fasting in itself, many followers turned to other ways of showing their love for God and atoning for sin. Fasting was not forgotten, but it was much less popular. The New Testament, for example, contains only a few references to it. Anna the prophetess was seen fasting and praying in the temple when Jesus was a boy, but that was a case of Jewish, not Christian, custom. After Christ died, the Apostles fasted on occasion. St. Paul, for instance, followed the examples before him, fasting after his conversion, before he began preaching.

But Christians generally had a different attitude about fasting. From the beginning, Christ had placed an emphasis on fasting as a means to make charity possible. Jesus stressed love of God and neighbor; fasting was a way of sacrificing to express that love, to free money and time to give to the poor. Christian theologians distinguish between Christian fasting and that of other religions. Noting that, among other things, Christians observe no taboos against eating certain foods (both Muslims and Jews avoid pork as unclean, for example), they suggest that the Christian custom is not really related to pagan practices of fasting. Nothing that God made should be refused because it is bad; everything that God created is good, they say. Christian fasting was simply man disciplining himself in the use of worldly goods to free them for other men. Theologians also stress the connection between fasting and prayer. Refraining from food was meant to free man for prayer, to concentrate and intensify his prayer by detaching him from worldly goods.

Although it was difficult to do because fasting is so simple a practice, the early Christians tried to make this distinction between themselves and the Jews around them. An early Christian writing, the *Didache*, told Christians to fast on Wednesdays and Fridays instead of on the Tuesdays and Thursdays on which Jews fasted. They set aside three seasons—during June, September, and December—as "ember weeks," dedicated to contemplation and spiritual renewal. On Wednesdays, Fridays, and Saturdays of those weeks, they fasted. Christians also made fast days periods of what they called "abstinence," meaning that meat and (sometimes) dairy foods were forbidden. Picking up the tradition of fasting as a preparation, Christians began fasting for one day before receiving God in the sacrament of Communion.

From this grew the tradition of a Lenten fast before Easter. Originally Lent was just a one-day vigil fast before the Easter communion. By the third century, the practice stretched to a two-day fast, at least, for this special feast. Some areas, notably in the eastern Mediterranean, were then fasting for the entire week before Easter. By the next century, Christians had decided to imitate the forty-day fasts of Moses and Jesus. That determination eventually eroded the true fast for Christians. When they realized what bodily harm they were causing, they gave it up and began an elaborate and constantly changing system of something they called "fasting," but that generally amounted only to taking less than the customary amount of food. At first they fasted until after Vespers (prayers) at sunset. The deadline shifted to about three o'clock in the afternoon, and then to noon itself. By the sixteenth century, breakfast was allowed. In the early part of this century, Roman Catholics took one full meal and two light meals during Lent; after 1966, they were obliged to keep that custom only on two days during Lent—Ash Wednesday and Good Friday.

They also abandoned the pre-Communion fast. When they stopped keeping a one-day vigil, they adopted the practice of fasting from midnight until they received Communion. In 1957, Pope Pius XII said Catholics could take any nonalcoholic liquid up until one hour before Communion. Later, all strictures were removed. The Anglican Church had similar rules, although most Christian churches have always left this practice up to the individual.

The Eastern Catholic rites and Eastern Orthodox churches have been a bit more faithful to fasting. At times they have kept up to one hundred-eighty days each year of at least partial fasts. Besides the traditional pre-Easter Lent, they observed the Lent of the Holy Apostles, from June 16 to 28, Mary's Lent, from August 1 to 14, and a Lent before Christmas, beginning November 15. Originally, only monks were obliged to fast, but church patriarchs charged the laity with fasting beginning in the eighth century. The practice has always varied widely, however, because local patriarchs or synods of bishops set customs.

Today, the fasting practices that remain in Christian churches are more varied than ever. Mormons, for example, are supposed to fast on the first Sunday of each month. They give the money saved by omitting meals to the poor. But most churches leave fasting to the individual, except when an immediate goal is at stake—then some churches will organize a specific fast. A few years ago many Christian churches organized day-long fasts to send aid to starving Biafrans. New Hampshire residents still celebrate an annual holiday, Fast Day, that was established in the seventeenth century as a plea to God to save their president, John Cutt. They no longer fast, but the holiday illustrates the onetime common practice of calling for a community fast among Christians.

Most Catholics are now left to follow their own conscience on fasting, and the prevailing belief is that there is some general obligation to do so. "The fact that fasting remains an integral part of Christian spirituality is underlined by Our Lord's saying that a certain kind of devil could be cast out 'only by prayer and fast' (Matthew 17:20). St. Paul listed fasting among the virtues of God's ministers (II Corinthians 6:5). Our Lord's own fasting set an example for all time," the Catholic journal *America* editorialized in its March 31, 1962 issue. Many of their popular saints—St. Francis of Assisi and St. Theresa of Avila among them—also provide examples. Only a few Catholic religious orders of nuns and priests still observe fasting rules: they are generally the contemplative orders whose members have left worldly life to devote themselves to prayer and penance in convents and monasteries.

HINDU FASTS

Among the world's five hundred million Hindus (belonging to many sects and schools), fasting can be a way of life. Hinduism cannot be described as easily as other religions; it has many gods, a well-developed mythology, and many beliefs that can easily be classified as mystical, magical, and superstitious. But it has no well-defined dogma. Formal liturgy and ritual, once an important part of Hinduism, have long since gone out of practice. Life itself is considered to be a "rite." Each person is responsible for his or her own salvation, and there is little distinction between the sacred and the earthly. In other words, every day is a sacred sabbath day because, more than in other religions, beliefs are supported by a way of life.

Ideally, Hindus lead their lives so that they are receptive to the faith and meaning that will then come to them. Meditation, prayer, seclusion, asceticism, and yoga exercises occupy much of a Hindu's time. Purity of mind and of body pervade the Hindu philosophy—both must be ever ready to unite with the Absolute, the supreme principle that is sometimes personified as Brahma. Hindus describe this union as an uplifting feeling of oneness with the universe. It is an experience to be desired as the ultimate Hindu goal. To achieve it, Hindus try to free themselves from desiring worldly goods.

Many practices can help induce union with the Absolute. One of them is fasting, because fasting purifies the body to a much higher degree than can be achieved in any other way. The various sects follow many different practices. One school adheres to a custom of taking less and less food in coordination with the waning of the moon. On the day of no moon, no food is consumed. Beginning with the next day, more and more food is eaten each day until a normal diet is consumed on the day of the full moon. Other Hindus go through a series of preparations each time they perform acts of personal worship, such as washings, avoidance of certain foods often culminating in a total fast, body postures and exercises, finger gestures, and breathing techniques. "There is no prayer without fasting" is a common Hindu expression Mahatma Gandhi was known to quote. He was always quick to add, however, that fasting in this instance means fasting of all the senses, not just abstinence from food.

Some Hindu sects put much more stock in the practice of yoga as a religious exercise, and they follow a much more rigorous yoga program. Yoga is a Sanskrit word meaning "union" or "unifying"; it signifies that yoga is a way to raise energy levels, to open oneself to the intense concentration that will bring on union with the divine Absolute. Yoga strengthens and purifies the body to make the union possible. Writing in *The Yoga of Health, Youth and Joy*, Sir Paul Dukes makes an unbeatable analogy: "An unsullied and spotless window of pure glass will admit light unhampered; a purified physique from which all toxic matter has been drastically eliminated is in a similar state. It does not have to do anything to function on a higher level, it merely has to be. This is the basic reason for fasting."

Although the length of the fasts has varied widely, fasting has always been a part of yoga. Historians believe yoga originated three or four thousand years ago among the people of the Himalayan mountains, who may have come to fasting by necessity. Living in such isolation, with so little opportunity to leave during the long, snowy winters, their food supplies must have grown short at times. Since reserves could not be replenished until spring, they were forced to fast.

In the East, yoga is considered a spiritual, mental, and physical regimen. True practitioners embrace yoga on all three levels as a means of improving the quality of life. In the West, however, where it is often not connected with religion, yoga is usually practiced merely as a physical routine to strengthen the body and improve health. This is called Hatha yoga, and many practitioners still fast as part of it; the aim remains self-mastery, even if the goal is now limited to strength and health. Hatha yoga schools usually tell their students to begin with a one-day fast, then to try fasting one day each week. Eventually they recommend a two-day fast. A few yoga authorities dispute these recommendations. They do not endorse fasting, arguing that eating a proper diet would create no need for cleansing the body of impurities.

OTHER RELIGIOUS FASTS

Hinduism, Christianity, Islam, and Judaism—each with distinct fasting traditions—are four of the six principal religions. Of the two others that complete the list, one believes in fasting, at least to a degree.

The man who first came to be called Buddha, "the enlightened one," was born a Hindu in the sixth century B.C. But he disputed some Hindu beliefs, notably the strict caste system that segregated classes of people and kept them in their stations for life. Although he broke with Hinduism, however, he kept the doctrine of recurring reincarnation, which held that each soul was always reborn as another creature. This, Buddha thought, was a fate worse than death. So he taught that attainment of *nirvana,* in which all desires had been extinguished, freed the soul from rebirth because all suffering resulted from desire. To reach his own state of *nirvana,* to become Buddha, he had lived a life of asceticism for six years. He practiced fasting and other deeds of self-mortification until he nearly wore himself to a skeleton. But later he decided that this extremism was not the way to reach nirvana. He preached that a "Middle Path" between the extremes of self-denial and self-indulgence could extinguish the desires and passions that precluded *nirvana.*

Only about 200,000 people today practice the sixth principal religion—Zoroastrianism. Leaders of this faith denounce fasting. They believe "fasting from evil" is much more important, and that fasting from food would be unnecessary if people committed no sins.

Interestingly, when a group called the Manicheans seceded from Zoroastrianism in the third century A.D., they returned to fasting as a means to goodness. They believe, as do other sects known collectively as Gnostics, that evil dominates good in all earthly matter. To liberate the goodness, Manicheans prayed, fasted, confessed to evil deeds, and sang hymns. They fasted each Sunday and during five two-day periods spread throughout the year. Between the fourth and fifth of these fasts, they imitated Islamic fasts, eating one small meal a day after sundown. An elite group of Manicheans fasted each Monday as well as Sunday, and kept the daily fast until sundown every day of the year. Manicheans are no more, however. They lived throughout the Roman Empire, North Africa, Spain, and the Mideast, but they were persecuted everywhere and were finally exterminated in the ninth century.

Among the other religious fasters are the Jainists, who also seceded from Hinduism. They take twelve vows, one of which is to fast on certain days. During the Middle Ages, a group in southern France called the Albigenses split from Christianity. Believing that all material things were evil, they committed suicide by starvation as the supreme religious act. In the Orient, there is some fasting among believers in Taoism. In China, a historical figure named Chang Ling became a national hero when, as a high government official in the third century B.C., he renounced his office and material goods and dedicated himself to the teachings of Lao Tzu, Taoism's founder. Very recently, anthropologists found a Christian cult in Mexico's Yucatan peninsula who claimed to "speak in tongues," as did Christ's apostles. Those who did said this miracle, speaking in one language and yet being understood by anyone who spoke any language, resulted from visions and trances induced by fasting.[1]

[1] Felicitas D. Goodman, Jeannette H. Henney, and Esther Pressel, *Trance, Healing, and Hallucination—Three Field Studies in Religious Experience* (New York: John Wiley & Sons, 1974).

5
political fasts

Golda Meir, G. Gordon Liddy, Simone Weil, Dick Gregory, convicted bank robber and Symbionese Liberation Army member Emily Harris, groups organized to fight hunger, British suffragettes, German terrorists, Bolivian dissidents, and the previously mentioned Terence MacSwiney and countless other Irish revolutionaries have all stopped eating at times for political reasons. They are just a few among many; this kind of fasting is also on the rise. Protestors usually employ fasting, or a hunger strike, as this tool is sometimes called, as a last resort. They are outsiders who cannot exert as much pressure in any other way. Protest fasting has occurred so frequently, in fact, that the medical world has taken up the subject as an ethical question—should the protestor be force-fed or be allowed to die?

Just because of that issue—the question of life itself and whether the establishment can and should bend a little to save a human life—protest fasting is a most effective weapon. As in other kinds of fasting, the origins of this political maneuver are lost. But the man who raised political fasting from a tactic to an art is unquestionably Mohandas Karamchand Gandhi, leader of India's independence movement. Never before or since has fasting been so effective politically. The British colonial government in India and officials back in England would literally cower each time the Mahatma, the "great soul," went on a protest fast. They feared anarchy if this beloved leader of so many millions of Indians were allowed to die. In 1930, the British viceroy there, Lord Irwin, reportedly even considered fasting as a counterattack, but he never did.

Gandhi was a cunning leader who was well acquainted with fasting before he used it politically (unlike many others who try it). Born into a Hindu family, Gandhi learned religion from his mother, who belonged to a sect that was strongly influenced by Islam. She taught him to be a vegetarian and to fast. Later, he fasted mainly for health reasons. Short and thin, he believed that food was merely medicine for the body, to be taken only in amounts needed for subsistence—certainly never too much. His weight proved that he practiced what he preached; it usually hovered around 100 pounds. In *Letters to a Disciple*, published notes he wrote to Madeleine Slade, an aristocratic Englishwoman who left her home and family to work with him in India and whom he called Mirabehn, he talked frequently about food and fasting. "An occasional fast and at least once per month is a good thing, it seems, even for lightweight people," he told her in January 1931. Earlier, in April 1929, he had written: "Always omit food when there is the slightest derangement in the digestive apparatus. Never mind the weakness. Strength will return when you are able to take food. But food itself will cause weakness, when the system cannot assimilate it."

As inspiration for his political fasts, Gandhi had only to look to his own antecedents. In the mid-1800s (Gandhi was born in 1869), a Hindu mystic named Ramakrishna fought to make India independent of the British. He helped the poor and once used fasting to push the British to make a few concessions to them. Ironically, it was the behavior of his fellow Indians and not the British that first prompted Gandhi to follow this example. In 1918, he was trying to mediate a labor dispute between British mill owners and ten thousand strikers in Ahmedabad who wanted a wage increase. Gandhi urged the workers to stand fast for a moderate increase but, when many began to starve, he heard complaints that he was not suffering as they were. Apparently acting on instinct, without giving it much thought, Gandhi vowed to stop eating until the workers got their raise. His first public fast worked wonders: the workers pleaded for forgiveness and some even volunteered to join him. The mill owners bent under the pressure and settled the dispute four days after Gandhi made his announcement. Fasting as part of Gandhi's campaign of passive resistance, or civil disobedience, had begun.

Again and again he would use this strategy to move India bit by bit toward unity and independence. On September 20, 1932, he started his most important fast. The British had prepared a plan for giving residents of India the right to vote that split caste Hindus, the Untouchables, Muslims, Europeans, and other groups into separate electorates. Gandhi had always fought to integrate the Untouchables into society, and he would not allow this outcast status to be conferred by the constitution, too. He announced he would hold out against the plan by fasting unto death. He wrote to Mirabehn: "There was no escape from it. It is both a privilege and a duty. It comes rarely to someone in a generation or generations. In nonviolence it is the crowning act."

Again it worked. Six days after it had begun, Gandhi broke the fast with a glass of orange juice. Britain had conceded—it would accept an alternative plan if the Hindus and Untouchables could agree to one. The Hindus relented, too. They opened their temples to the Untouchables, ate with them, and put together an agreement that Britain approved. "For the first time Gandhi had imposed his will on a British government," writes Geoffrey Ashe in his book, *Ghandi*. "When the entire fabric of nationalism was crumbling, he had halted the Imperial trend toward fragmentation and demoralization. He might or might not have achieved the same political end without fasting. At least the fast gave urgency. . . . Untouchability was not dead, but it would never be the same. An India going to pieces under pressure had pulled itself together and again had a moral advantage over its masters."

This greatest of fasts illustrates a point that has often been left out of tales about Mahatma Gandhi. He fasted to drive the various segments of Indian society together and to do penance for their violence and rioting as often as he did to pressure the British. Without stirring Indian consciences, he could probably never have achieved what he did.

Gandhi fasted again many times before he was struck down at the age of seventy-eight by an assassin's bullet. He was always cautious and careful, spacing his fasts so that his body could recover in between. He knew that a lifetime of fasting and health had enabled him to go without food as others could not. He recognized its power in an August 1933 letter to Mirabehn: "Eat your food thankfully and keep yourself fit for service. Time for you may come when you might have to take up a similar fast. Under certain circumstances it is the one weapon which God has given us for use in times of utter helplessness."

Great Britain finally agreed to give India its independence in 1947, but Gandhi's fasts were not yet over. The Muslim minority wanted its own nation, fearing domination by the Hindus if they did not separate. Gandhi wanted a united, secular India; he urged that Muslims be endowed with some powers. Britain decided to let the two groups split territory into what became India and Pakistan. But some Muslims were dispersed throughout India, and Gandhi wanted to assure that they had rights. In January 1948 he started his last fast, one to stir the Hindus to acknowledge rights of Muslims. The Mahatma was now very weak, and the prodding did its job very quickly; Hindus worked to present a plan to him, and five days into the fast he broke it. Several days later, however, Hindu extremists killed him.

Through this entire period, many other Indian leaders, including Jawaharlal Nehru, later to become the country's first prime minister, followed his example and fasted. But none could get such results.

The political fast is always a tricky strategy. It may work or it may backfire or it may not do anything. Gandhi's fasts succeeded because he was morally upright, his cause was just, his timing was good, his followers were many and ardent, and his goals were concrete, attainable, and important. His fasts succeeded on such a grand scale because all those elements combined to enable Gandhi to capture the world's attention and support. Lack of any of those elements does not necessarily mean failure. But it surely means more muted success.

Have you, for example, ever heard of Danilo Dolci? English novelist and critic Aldous Huxley once called him "the Gandhi of Sicily." For more than a quarter of a century, Dolci has been fighting poverty and crime there. Using public fasting and other forms of protest, he has taken on the unresponsive national Italian government as well as local governments, supposedly Mafia-controlled, that ignore or bilk the Sicilian peasants and keep them in poverty. Dolci first turned to fasting after he was arrested in 1952 for rounding up unemployed fishermen to finish an abandoned road project—without getting official permission to build the road. Later he fasted to protest delays in construction of a government dam, one Sicilians needed to provide water for farming the arid land. He has had other successes since then, enough to win him a nomination for the Nobel Peace Prize. He is certainly a local hero. But Dolci is aiming at an abstract, moving target. Whatever good the social reformer has done cannot win him the acclaim that Gandhi drew. That is not to dismiss what good Dolci has done as unimportant, but merely to illustrate the different results that fasting can bring.

The British suffragettes used fasting to their benefit, too. And they certainly attracted attention in England. The world's first feminist manifesto flowed from the mind and pen of an English governess in 1792. That is when Mary Wollstonecraft, who was also the mother of *Frankenstein*'s author, Mary Shelley, published *A Vindication of the Rights of Women*. But more than one hundred years later, women in England had still not budged more than an inch toward winning the vote. After 1906, when seven suffrage bills went down to defeat in Parliament, and for the next several years, the suffragettes turned militant. They protested and were arrested and put in prison. To win political sympathy, they also fasted during imprisonment. Sympathy they got. The government looked cruel, especially when they began force-feeding those who went on extended fasts. Finally, in 1913, the government tried a new tack. Parliament passed the Prisoners Temporary Discharge for Ill Health Act, better known as the "Cat and Mouse Act." It allowed law enforcement officials to release fasting women from prison, only to rearrest and reimprison them each time they got their strength back. This happened again and again until 1918, when Englishwomen at last won the right to vote.

Over the years, the British government has had to cope with protest fasters many times. Perhaps the most exasperating have been the Irish militants. There has been tension between Ireland and England since the twelfth century, when the Roman Catholic Pope gave Ireland to the King of England. Both countries were Catholic at the time, however, so there were few real problems. The situation grew worse when King Henry VIII left Catholicism. The Irish thought his split with the Church voided his right to rule Ireland. They've been fighting England ever since. They seem to have taken to protest fasting as a duck does to water. Their deep-rooted faith, with its history of persecutions and martyrs, has apparently convinced them that it is perfectly acceptable, even admirable, to give their life to rid their country of illegitimate Protestant rulers. First it was practically a whole island of fasters, such as Mayor Terence MacSwiney of Cork. Since the Ireland Act of 1920, which split the island in two and gave the southern three-fourths its independence, the protest has been concentrated among the Catholics in the north. Typical are four members of the Irish Republican Army who went on a hunger strike during their trial for setting off bombs in London in 1973. Other IRA members joined them in sympathy. Eventually, most stopped when they got some concession, transfer to another prison, movement out of solitary confinement, or visitation rights, for example), but one man died in 1974 after sixty-five days without food. Many, many other IRA members have fasted over the years; they are tough and militant, and they get encouragement from their supporters.

Ironically, the Irish government itself recently has had to cope with protest fasters, on occasion from terrorists. A most amusing case, however, was reported in the *New York Times* in May, 1978. Three leaders in Tuam, a fifteen-hundred-year-old town with six thousand residents in west central Ireland, decided to go on a hunger strike after the state-owned railway said it would stop freight train service and the state-owned sugar company announced it would shut one of its two plants there. Fearing that the two decisions would destroy their town economically, the three political rivals joined in the fast. Eight days later they had won; Dublin relented and reversed itself.

Hunger-striking prisoners often cause authorities the most problems; they are put in the position of force-feeding the fasters, who usually resist violently. Some governments, such as England's, have just given up on the very determined. After being told by a doctor what they can expect to happen, the prisoners are left to decide for themselves. Germany has chosen the other course. A few years ago, leaders of the terrorist Baader-Meinhof gang began fasting in their Stuttgart prison cells before their trial for the 1972 bombing murders of four U.S. servicemen, thirty-four attempted killings, arson, and bank robbery. Perhaps because

Germany has been very sensitive about its law enforcement activities since Nazi activities during World War II, authorities decided three weeks after the fasting began that they would not allow the terrorists to die. They began force-feeding, tying, taping, and holding down the prisoners when necessary. If a prisoner is cooperative, he will receive nourishment through a tube in his mouth. But, if he resists, he must be fed by a tube through his nose, a painful process that sometimes had to be stretched over three hours to avoid causing vomiting and kidney damage. For months the terrorists received an 1,800-calorie diet through tubes every day.

Eventually, the terrorists quit their strike. But when they were found guilty in court, they started fasting anew. Last year, they broke the fast four days before their colleagues kidnapped top West German industrialist Hanns-Martin Schleyer. The kidnappers asked for the prisoners' release in exchange for Schleyer, so the terrorists apparently began eating to gain strength in preparation. That was not to be. Eventually, the imprisoned terrorists committed suicide and Schleyer was found dead.

Almost at the opposite end of the spectrum from these German terrorists are the people who fast en masse to end world hunger. They do not believe the conclusions of a recent Congressional report warning that future generations would face mass starvation unless nations began to control populations or the world drastically increased its production of food (although they do not deny that those measures would be helpful and worthwhile aims). There is a third choice, they say: people, particularly Americans, can change the way they eat. If the gap between the rich, too-high-protein meals that are customary in moneyed areas and the scrappy, high-carbohydrate diet of poor peoples and nations were smaller, starvation and malnutrition would not have to exist. Too much effort, they say, goes to provide too few people with too rich food. Many poor countries even export food their own people should be eating because they need the cash. And too many rich nations waste food; that could be stopped.

Many groups have fasted to dramatize this situation. Some have already been mentioned in connection with religious fasting. There are others. In 1974, the U.S. Senate passed a resolution setting aside November 24 of that year as a "National Day of Fasting," and as a period to reassess the American way of life. Groups such as Bread for the World, Project F.A.S.T., World Vision International, and the Committee for Creative Non-Violence have all advocated similar days of fasting.

Most recently, Werner Erhard's est Foundation started its Hunger Project, aimed at ending starvation by 1997. In its promotional brochure, which states that "each year fifteen million people die whose deaths would otherwise not occur were it not for hunger. Three quarters of these people are children. In addition, at least four hundred million people are seriously undernourished." The Hunger Project says there is enough food to feed the world's population. It asked everyone to fast on November 14, 1977 and on the fourteenth of every month thereafter to raise money and save food for the cause. The project says that this will create the right climate for a transformation in eating habits. They might as well have been listening to Mahatma Gandhi, who wrote to Mirabehn forty-five years ago: ". . . the full-mealers deprive their neighbor of their portion. God's economy provides from day to day just enough food for all in just medicinal doses. We are all of the tribe of full-mealers. Instinctively to know the medicinal dose required is a Herculean task, for by parental training we are gluttons."

What about the others mentioned at the beginning of this chapter? They are just a small sampling of fasters with a cause. Shortly after World War II, Israel's future prime minister, Golda Meir, led a four-day hunger strike protesting the refusal of Britain to allow Jewish refugees to land in Palestine, then under British control. G. Gordon Liddy led a different hunger strike. In August 1977, when Liddy was still behind bars at Allenwood Prison for masterminding the Watergate break-in, he fasted and encouraged his fellow inmates to fast for five days to protest prison food, inmate job assignments, and working conditions. For his troubles, Liddy was transferred from minimum-security Allenwood to the tougher, maximum-security Lewisburg Prison. About six weeks earlier, Liddy had gone on a twenty-four-hour fast against living conditions at Allenwood and an order to take down a homemade partition in a prisoner's cell.

Emily Harris was lonely. The Symbionese Liberation Army member, who is also connected with the Hearst kidnapping, went on a thirty-four-day fast in 1977 to protest being kept in solitary confinement during her eleven-years-to-life sentence for a robbery conviction. Harris dropped 25 pounds from her 108-pound frame, but was still in isolation when she resumed eating. French writer Simone Weil starved herself to death when the movement resisting the Nazi occupation during World War II would not allow her to go on a risky, critical mission. In late 1977, about twelve hundred students, religious leaders, journalists, workers, and relatives joined in a hunger strike to demand the release of and blanket amnesty for Bolivia's political prisoners. Twenty days into the strike, Bolivia's president Hugo Banzer ordered police to begin arresting the fasters; but Banzer relented the next day, released the fasters, and declared a general amnesty for political prisoners.

Then there is Dick Gregory. The Vietnam war brought Gregory to fasting. He was a well-known, popular comedian and civil rights activist in 1967, when he decided to pick up Mahatma Gandhi's weapon to draw attention to what was going on in Southeast Asia and to protest United States involvement. At that time, much of America was ambivalent about the war. Gregory knew how to get mileage from his fast; he knew how to use the media. He called a press conference to announce his action, choosing the period between Thanksgiving and Christmas to go without food. He put a $1,000 bond in the hands of two Chicago journalists in case anyone wanted to try to prove he didn't keep his fast. And he kept a full schedule during the period, doing nightclub gigs, television shows, college lectures, and plenty of traveling between them. When Christmas came, the comedian decided to keep going; he did not break the fast until New Year's Day, 1968.

Of course, Gregory's fast did not make the United States quit Vietnam, but it did help raise the public consciousness about the war. It also got Gregory hooked on fasting; he has used it again and again to protest on a variety of issues—the problems of American Indians, the misdirection of the police in enforcement of drug laws in going after drug addicts instead of pushers, South Africa's policy of apartheid, world hunger—and to get himself out of jail on a couple of occasions.

Fasting also raised Gregory's consciousness. It effected a profound change on his lifestyle, making him extremely aware of what and how much he ate and prompting him to go back to the athletic regimen he had practiced in his younger days. Gregory may have started fasting as a protest, but that's not where it ended. He now fasts for health reasons. And anyone who wants a strong argument for fasting for health should take a long look at Gregory's before and after photographs. He turned from a pudgy, paunchy man into a slim, trim one who looks much younger than his age. Of course, fasting alone could not have done that, but what it precipitated did.

6
to your health?

Doughnuts or a danish for breakfast, fast-food fare for lunch, porkchops, home-fried potatoes, peas, and cherry pie for dinner—add a candy bar, an apple, or a couple of packaged snack foods, soda pop, a can of beer, and lots of coffee, and you have the equivalent of a typical daily American meal plan. Too much sugar, salts, fats, additives, and preservatives make the diets we eat unhealthy, although there may be nothing wrong with any one food. Now think about the environment in which most of us live; there is too much air and water pollution, and many of those pollutants (lead and mercury, for example) find their way into the foods we eat. When you also consider that we get too little fresh air, sunshine, and exercise and that many of us smoke cigarettes, you can conclude that the American way of life is not a healthy one. If the Industrial Revolution and the progress it brought had not taken place, things might be different; but in today's world, if you want to be healthy, you have to work at it.

Most people who fast for their health try to eat well and exercise, but they feel that that is not enough. Some pollutants and additives cannot be avoided. During normal times, the body works to eliminate some impurities, which fasters like to call toxins, or "poisons." But it cannot put a great deal of its available energy into cleaning out its digestive system if the system is being used constantly. They compare that to, say, the cleaning staff at the office; it doesn't come in during the day, when people are working, but at night, when no one is there.

Like Dick Gregory, many people who fast for their health come to it for other reasons—protesting, dieting, religion, or self-discipline. Others pick it up from friends or because they have decided intellectually that the body needs to rest once in a while, just as everything else does. Recently, many runners have become fasting zealots. They first tried fasting as training for a race, as part of a depletion-carbohydrate reloading regimen to increase stamina, then stayed when they convinced themselves it had health benefits.

Those who do fast for their health usually feel good when they fast. Listen to some typical comments from them.

"I can just feel my body changing, and I know from that feeling that fasting is a very healthy thing to do."

"I feel so alert when I fast."

"It really changes your attitudes about food. You can go into a fast loving potato chips and soda and pizza, but when you finish one you only want to put good foods into your body."

"I fast when I feel bogged down. It makes me feel very independent, very much in control of myself. I don't need as much sleep and yet I feel calm, not at all anxious."

"I fast purely for health reasons, not because I believe it's a mystical phenomenon. But some things that happen can be interpreted as mystical—it allows me to have other than normal perceptions and feelings, maybe because the body is not clogged up. They tell you you get euphoric, and I do feel a bit high."

"I have a much different image of my body when I fast. I lose weight, and I feel good in it."

Those comments come from men and women who have gone without food for from twenty-four hours to twenty-seven days. Many are repeaters who fast for ten days or seven days at regular intervals. Some fast whenever the spirit moves them. As you can see for yourself, the health benefits they claim are—for the most part—intangible (except for losing weight, the subject of the next chapter). They are not unimportant, and will be discussed later in this chapter. But you may have heard more extraordinary claims about the benefits of fasting, namely, that it can cure and even prevent disease. Those theories belong to another group of fasters, who are much more positive about what fasting can do. They have the most complete philosophy about fasting, and they call themselves "natural hygienists."

NATURAL HYGIENE

"It's a revolutionary and drastic change we are asking for," says Werner Kist, "it's like Columbus finding out the world is flat. . . . The hygienic system really bucks society." Kist is president of the Chicago chapter of the American Natural Hygiene Society, Inc. (ANHS). From its national headquarters office in a residential Chicago neighborhood, the thirty-year-old organization promotes "natural hygiene" as a way of life. It disbelieves modern medical theories and therapies. In their place it substitutes ideas prevalent before modern medicine was born. Natural hygienists believe in the "holistic" approach to health—a prevention theory that they say emphasizes the functional and organic relationships among the physical, mental, spiritual, and psychological parts of the body, and treats all the parts as well as the whole. In less obscure terms, the ANHS way of life means a vegetarian diet, consumption of only natural, nonprocessed foods and distilled water (which the society sells), lots of sleep and rest, abstention from coffee, tea, cigarettes, and liquor, plenty of fresh air, sunshine, and exercise, natural childbirth, and control of emotions.

There is nothing revolutionary or reactionary about that. But another tenet may startle. They do not believe in medicine, inoculations, or other drugs. They do not believe in the germ theory of disease, a basic medical doctrine that states that infections, contagious diseases, and some other ailments are caused by viruses and bacteria. In their eyes, French physician Louis Pasteur is an imposter and his theory is a hoax. "The doctor of the future will give no medicine, but will interest his patients in the care of the human frame and diet, and the cause and prevention of disease," says a quote at the bottom of a society brochure. The words come not from a quack, but from (they say) Thomas A. Edison.

Without medicine, when a natural hygienist gets sick, there is only one way to recuperate: fast. The theory is that in fasting, the body can rest from most of its essential duties and concentrate on healing itself. Whatever the disease—cancer, cold, arthritis, anemia, tumors, diabetes, ulcers, asthma, tuberculosis, epilepsy, migraine headaches, appendicitis, eczema, insomnia, heart disease, gallstones, polio, hypertension (high blood pressure), allergies, goiter, hay fever, hemorrhoids, colitis, or you name it, because the list could go on forever—fasting in the therapy.

Have you ever hear the old joke that has a patient asking, "Doc, how long will it take to cure my cold?" "Well," the doctor replies, "about two weeks with the medicine I just gave you and about a fortnight without it."

The joke just about epitomizes what natural hygienists believe, except not just for the cold, which has stubbornly resisted any medicine so far invented. They say the body will take care of most ailments itself if it can direct all its energies to the trouble spot. They do not claim that fasting itself cures a disease but, instead, that it allows the body to heal itself.

Although the society began around thirty years ago, its roots go back much further. In Europe, natural hygiene as a healing art may be traced at least to the eighteenth century. Some members say hygiene evolved from hydropathy, a therapy once popular in Germany that used enemas, drinking water, washings, special showers, and other water-related ideas to cure illness. Theoretically, hygienists combined the best of hydropathy with the practice of eating only natural foods and the belief that the body cures itself if given the chance. Hygienists are much more clear about their American genealogy. Their theories came from Sylvester Graham, the man who invented the graham cracker and pioneered the use of whole wheat flour. Graham combed the country during the 1880s preaching dietary reform and healthful living, including clothing reform for women who wore the popular tightly laced corsets and high-heeled, pointy-toed shoes.

In the ANHS theory of disease, unhealthful living habits, not microscopic "bugs," cause illness. If you do not get enough sleep, or if you fail to exercise, you will eventually get sick. If you dine on greasy, prepared foods that are loaded with chemical additives, you will get sick. Any departure from good hygiene principles will lead to enervation, which means the body lacks adequate nerve energy and vitality, or toxemia, which means poisons have spread throughout the body. Most acute illness can be traced to imperfect digestion—intestinal toxemia. But that is not the only kind of toxemia; when the body dissolves its old and unhealthy tissue, the theory goes, the waste, which contains toxins, is not always eliminated by the body. People keep interfering with the cleansing process. Disease is "evidence of the system's failure to keep clean, and with reasonable care is preventable," says one brochure. When the body gets sick, it is rejecting the human lifestyle and trying to effect reform.

Hygienists believe the body will cure itself, under two conditions. First, you have to remove the cause: stop eating the wrong foods, start getting exercise, air, and sun, and begin practicing the other principles of good health. Second, because the body has only so much energy available for its vital daily functions (digestion, circulation, respiration, and so on) and for healing, you have to go on a fast. Fasting conserves some energy that normally fuels body functions, freeing it for the body to use to cure itself. Thus fasting "is more than just not eating," explains Mark Huberman, the society's current national president. Ideally, a fast means giving the body the most complete rest possible: stop eating, drink only pure, demineralized water, stay in bed, do as little reading, talking, walking, watching television, and everything else as possible. Any extra activity reduces the benefits of a fast, and the best results come when a person fasts "until completion," that is, when hunger returns.

Fasting can also be preventive medicine. "We use fasting toward healing, repairing, restoring and rejuvenating the body," Huberman says. The word "rejuvenation" keeps cropping up in talks with natural hygienists. By it they mean that as the body is fasted, it almost becomes younger, it is revitalized. During a fast, the body consumes its fat stores and some lean tissue. When eating resumes, the body replaces the lean tissue it lost with new cells. Thus, with a higher number of new cells than before, the body is, in a way, reborn. Ideally, ANHS suggests, everyone should fast one day each week to prevent small problems from brewing into full-fledged ailments. Fasting is the first step on the road to proper living. "Once you give your body a breather (by fasting) you've got to get back to the right regimen," Huberman insists.

ANHS puts a great deal of distance between itself and today's battery of health and food faddists. One member tells with much amusement the story of a publisher who approached another member, proposing that he write a book about the currently popular liquid protein fasts. An ANHS member would never consider such a thing; the very idea goes against the society's grain. Its members have little patience with people who search for health by skipping merrily from megavitamin therapy to vegetarian diet, from practicing yoga to jogging, with each phase lasting little more than a few weeks, and all the while smoking cigarettes. They disdain people who are not hygiene-for-life believers. An ANHS member is in this society, and lifestyle, for all of his or her days.

TRUE BELIEVERS

Even if they don't always live up to practicing all their principles, most ANHS members are true believers. Many came to natural hygiene and fasting after a personal experience with an ailment that modern medicine could not cure. Most others became believers after learning of such cases, often from a relative or close friend. Huberman's story illustrates both. Now in his mid-twenties, he appears to be the picture of American success, not the type you would cast in the role of president of a society labeled "anti-scientific." Bright and articulate, the techniques he learned as a theater major in college shine through in his personality. He later went to law school, and now practices in Youngstown, Ohio. He was brought up in hygiene; his father turned to it when he was stricken with polio and his mother tried it when she had appendicitis. His father now travels the country giving health lectures. His parents owned a health food store long before they became a national fad. When members elected Huberman a member of the national board before he celebrated his nineteenth birthday, Huberman became the youngest member ever to serve the society in any official capacity. He is by far the youngest president.

He also claims to have used fasting successfully as therapy. After his second year of law school, Huberman popped his eardrum on an airplane flight to California. He could no longer hear in one ear. Medical doctors do not have a "cure" for this. They may have replaced the living tissue with a plastic eardrum and prescribed antibiotics to kill any accompanying infection. An infection can disturb the body's balancing mechanism, also located in the ear, and can also spread to the brain. Indeed, when Huberman consulted an ear, nose and throat specialist, the doctor did give him a prescription for an antibiotic.

But Huberman also went to see the licensed chiropractor who is vice-president of the ANHS board, D.J. Scott. Scott runs a health institute in Cleveland. He reminded Huberman that fasting would help heal and restore the eardrum. Although Huberman admits he is a terrible faster who has great difficulty doing nothing, he took Scott's advice.

"It was frustrating as hell, being in bed doing nothing," he says. "You ask what you are doing for yourself, and the answer seems to be nothing."

On the sixth day, he returned to consult with the physician. Although Huberman says he had not taken any of the antibiotics the specialist had prescribed or any other medication, the doctor told him he was recovering. The antibiotics were working, he said.

Chuckling, Huberman went home and continued fasting for five more days. By then he was completely healed, he claims; his hearing was restored.

Huberman's story is trivial compared to others that hygienists tell. An ANHS past president named Jack Goldstein can relate a more dramatic tale. He does so in a book titled *Triumph Over Disease—By Fasting and Natural Diet*. Goldstein, a Doctor of Podiatric Medicine who now practices in Livonia, Michigan, says he was close to death in 1964. Goldstein was suffering from ulcerative colitis. After six years of drugs, doctors told him it was time to remove surgically the trouble spots—his entire large intestine and rectum. For the rest of his life, he would have had to eliminate bodily wastes through a bag attached to his abdomen. Instead of facing the surgery and the routine that followed, he fasted for six weeks, under the supervision of a doctor. He claims that the fast, later accompanied by a vegetarian diet, worked. Goldstein has gotten a lot of publicity; his area, near Detroit, now boasts the largest ANHS chapter.

Total membership is still tiny; only three thousand annually pay a "contribution" of between $10 and $100 to join. But another seven thousand pay to subscribe to the ANHS magazine. The nonprofit, tax-exempt society also publishes about thirty paperback books on natural hygiene and fasting and distributes another one hundred titles. Recently sales are up, so more money is coming in, and a member who died a short time ago left ANHS a bequest. With the new funds, Huberman wants to advertise, to build membership, and to make educational films—in short, to spread the word.

If the society recognizes one factor that can limit membership, it is that ANHS has only seven "approved" hygienists (most of whom are chiropractors) throughout the country. Medical doctors, members say, should treat only bone breaks, fractures, wounds that need stitches, and other physical problems. Many members, paradoxically, also consult doctors for a diagnosis, which is theoretically unnecessary to hygienists. But members need someone trained in supervising fasts to watch over them when they are sick. Huberman plans to increase the number of hygienists somehow. After all, he sums up, "Our position is if hygiene can't help you, nothing will."

MEDICAL REACTION

A drug, a treatment, or a therapy with that kind of potential could win the Nobel prize in medicine and reap billions of dollars. Only a few miles from the ANHS headquarters, the American Medical Association has its own national office in a downtown Chicago high rise. AMA dismisses the idea of any such panacea, let alone that it could incorporate fasting. To almost every medical doctor, fasting as therapy for anything but weight reduction in the grossly overweight is nothing more than antiscientific heresy. Medicine and medical therapy are founded on scientific proof, doctors say. Does ANHS have any?

No, ANHS cannot prove—scientifically or otherwise—that fasting is therapeutic. "We don't have any documentation," Chicago chapter president Kist admits. Kist blames the lack of proof on different beliefs among the practitioners. "They don't agree on the little things," he says. Some feel you should fast once a week, others think it should be done only when needed, and still others say fasting must be done for at least a week or two to give the body time to adjust and to make the change worthwhile.

Fasting proponents make the most headway in convincing people that fasting works by using the testimonial, the oldest and often the most effective form of advertisement. Stories such as

Jack Goldstein's reach people on an emotional level and can make many converts.

That in itself is enough to make medical doctors and consumer protectionists wary. "The testimonial is used very often by a quack who has no scientific training or evidence that his therapy works," says Stephen Barrett, M.D., coeditor of *The Health Robbers—How to Protect Your Money and Your Life*, a book that discusses some current medical frauds. That book did not include mention of fasting, however. "There are thousands of these big and little methods—it would be an endless task to do them all," says Barrett, who practices psychiatry in Allentown, Pennsylvania. But, without knowing much about the ANHS, Barrett mentioned two other practices that should make a cautious person wonder about the validity of a therapy.

- Billing it as a panacea, a cure-all, that works on any and all ailments.
- Quoting obscure references as proof of respectability.

Indeed, ANHS fails both tests. Its members say repeatedly that fasting and natural hygiene work on anything (although some leave themselves an escape hatch by saying that fasting to completion is necessary; many people quit before the point when hunger returns). Second, believers do quote obscure sources. A book ANHS distributes called *Therapeutic Fasting*, by Arnold DeVries, mentions several "doctors" by name without mentioning where most can be located, for example. The ANHS book list also carries notice of a 106-page "historic" speech delivered by Russell T. Trall before the Smithsonian Institution in the 1860s. Trall may very well have given the speech, but the Smithsonian cannot confirm it. Its records from those years have been destroyed by fire.

Barrett and other doctors are quick to point out that many believers in fraudulent therapies are not malevolent; they actually believe in what they advocate. Therapeutic fasting seems to be that kind of quackery. There is little money to be made by the society, and there are too few hygiene practitioners to be making millions by bilking innocent patients. And much of what hygienists preach—exercise, fresh air, fresh foods, sunshine—is worthwhile.

For their part, hygienists counter that medical doctors have little training in nutrition and do not understand fasting. In fact, many medical schools offer only minimal instruction in nutrition.

(Many licensed nutritionists and dieticians have agreed that too few doctors know enough about nutrition, and that even fewer actually keep up with changes in the field.) ANHS members challenge doctors to examine some of their cases and explain them.

Actually, there are many reasons why fasting could appear to work as therapy. Some diseases and ailments can be "cured" or at least mitigated merely by losing weight, so that as a faster drops pounds, he or she feels better. High blood pressure and arthritis fall into this category. Some children with epilepsy have been treated for short periods by feeding them a diet that creates ketones (see chapter 8). Fasting also induces the formation of ketones, and that could bring a temporary feeling of well-being to epileptics. Ulcers, diarrhea, allergies, and other diseases that may be affected by the foods we eat or do not eat could also appear to be cured by fasting.

In many experiments over the years, people given sugar pills, vitamins, or fake pills when they think they are receiving medicine say they get better and sometimes actually do get better just because they think they should be getting well. This phenomenon, called the placebo effect, can also work with fasting; if they believe it will work, it appears to. Emotions often play a large part in causing symptoms of disease. (You may now be picturing the middle-aged housewife who is a hypochondriac, but this is actually more common than that.) When emotions work to cause or aggravate an illness, they can also work to dispel some symptoms.

Willing a cure may also be at work among fasters. Sometimes persons with incurable diseases keep themselves alive simply by refusing to die. Some people with physical problems or handicaps want to get well so much and work so hard at it that they make more progress than seemed possible to the medical world. On a different level, this may be working among believers in therapeutic fasting.

Perhaps the most important factor to be considered when analyzing people who have been "cured" by fasting is that most diseases are self-limiting. Doctors say that in 60 to 80 percent of all ailments, given time, the body will heal itself. But fasting has nothing to do with it; it cannot speed recovery by allowing the body to concentrate its energy. In fact, fasting may be detrimental, may actually slow recovery because it deprives the body of food protein needed to replace unhealthy tissue.

Doctors zero in on protein and mineral loss as their biggest complaint about fasting for any reason. Dehydration may also become a problem. They warn older people not to immobilize themselves by staying in bed, lest they harm their bones, which lose calcium. And, as in all quackeries, they disapprove because a sick person does not seek real help, but wastes sometimes precious time with a fraudulent therapy.

LESSER HEALTH CLAIMS

But the fact that fasting cannot work miracles does not mean that it has no health value. For some reason it has attracted many devotees over the years. Recently, as rich, famous, and glamorous jet-set types have adopted it, fasting has also acquired a certain cachet. Yet it is impossible to make definite statements about what fasting can absolutely do for you. It may only improve your mental health, your mental image of yourself. It still gets very mixed reviews when all sides are considered, and most doctors clearly and firmly disapprove. No medical research has been conducted on these aspects of fasting. There are no statistics, no data. What follows is all pure reporting, rather like the testimonials doctors warn about when they talk about quackery.

For some people, nothing makes them feel as refreshed as getting out of a long, warm shower, donning a well-pressed set of new clothes, and going out into a fresh, clear, crisp day. Fasting advocates compare their feelings after a short "housecleaning" fast to that kind of sensation. Generally, your liver, kidneys, skin, and excretory system remove impurities and wastes from your body. They do not always do a perfect job, although they do a good one. Even if nothing is coming in through your digestive system, the cleansing organs keep working. Then the body can, for example, flush out the intestines, particularly if you drink plenty of water. It will probably also remove other wastes that may not be released as readily when the body is more occupied. But it does not clear out all other substances that have been proven to be or may be harmful. Some people, for example, think they can lower their blood cholesterol and fat levels by fasting. That does happen for a short time on a fast, but cholesterol levels vary from day to day anyhow. If you eat nothing containing cholesterol on any day or eat much less containing it, but continue to eat other foods, your cholesterol level will go down. So fasting produces no great benefits in this area. And once the body begins to metabolize fats for fuel, most fasters show an increase in cholesterol and triglyceride levels.

The verdict on the theory that fasting cleans out chemical food additives has not yet come in. Unfortunately, medical authorities do not yet know enough about the way the body handles all additives. If any are stored, doctors believe they most likely would be excreted during a twenty-four-hour fast. Some food dyes may be metabolized by the body. If so, there is no way to tell when and if they will be eliminated during a fast.

Many fasters think they are ridding the body of wastes because of a whitish coating they get on their tongue after several days of fasting and because of the bad breath that accompanies the coating. It smells bad enough to suggest that toxic substances are being released inside. This is not so; the coating and the bad breath accompany a process called ketogenesis, in which fat tissue is turned into fuel for the body.

Doctors believe these ketones, produced during ketogenesis, cause the euphoric "high" some people experience during a fast of more than five or six days. Fasters have long touted this high as a reason for fasting. The sense of well-being can be almost as strong as a drug-induced high. This euphoria usually does not last too long, but neither does it come to a crashing, intolerable end.

More than by this ketone-induced high, fasters are sometimes elated by the feeling of independence from food and control of their own bodies. Feelings of power and endurance can be terribly important, especially to people who think they have little control over many day-to-day activities. Runners express the same satisfaction and feeling of accomplishment. In fact, most such acts of discipline create it. What is more, fasting, because eating is often considered to be an involuntary action, can bring double gratification to those who are not happy with their eating habits. Boredom, anxiety, guilt, unhappiness, and many other emotions often prompt a person to eat. If a person who is very vulnerable to eating binges triggered by emotion can complete a period of fasting, he or she feels enormous power.

Sometimes this power can also be translated to a permanent change in eating habits. Once a person sees that he or she can eat rationally—can resist the temptation to go on a binge—that person can begin to use self-restraint to stick with a sensible, unemotional eating regimen. The simplest, most obvious comparison that comes to mind is alcoholism or drug addiction, and they do share symptoms with emotional eating. Alcoholics and drug addicts must learn to give up their habit for good, however, which a "foodaholic" (and they are not necessarily overweight people) cannot do. But one clean break with food can effect a change in attitude toward food. It can reduce dependency on food when emotion makes the foodaholic crave it.

Most of us eat too much food. Have you noticed how groggy or sleepy you get after a heavy meal? You are not necessarily tired, just lackadaisical. Some people have been aware of this phenomenon for a long time. Henry IV of France hinted at it in the sixteenth century when he said, "Great eaters and great sleepers are incapable of anything else that is great." Some fasters have found that the converse is true: if they fast they are more alert. Fasting drags them out of sluggishness. This usually works only on a short fast, because fasting slows metabolism and eventually weakens the body.

Some people even claim fasting brings a certain mental clarity and stimulates creativity. Their awareness is heightened, they say. Upton Sinclair, author of *The Jungle* and perhaps the best known of the muckrakers who crusaded against America's social and economic ills at the beginning of this century, believed this to be true. (Sinclair was always a food faddist, however, and he blithely switched from diet to diet everytime a new one caught his fancy. He was enthralled with fasting, and even wrote a book about its therapeutic value, *The Fasting Cure*, in 1911. And something aroused Sinclair's creativity; by the time he died at the age of ninety, he had written ninety books and thousands of magazine articles and pamphlets.) If fasting releases a person from thoughts about food, it could enable that person to concentrate on a higher level. But most of us find that we think about food constantly during a fast, if only because we cannot isolate ourselves from the rest of the world.

What about fasting's much-vaunted reputation as a fountain of youth? Will your body really be rejuvenated as old cells dissolve to be replaced by new ones? Hardly. Fasting will probably make you look older, not younger. Skin dries out when it is not getting enough fat. Just as tanned skin will eventually look older because it has been dried out, so will the skin of someone who fasts repeatedly. Fasting can also make you lose color, and gray is old. And when weight is lost too rapidly, facial muscles do not have time to adjust, and that can also make you look older.

Inside your body, the skeleton bears most of the burdens of age. True aging involves more loss than gain of calcium by the bones. Bones then shrink, become brittle, and are more susceptible to fracture. Calcium is lost during a fast, and whether all of it is always regained is uncertain. So fasting has either a neutral or a detrimental effect on aging.

RUNNING AND FASTING

Runners—both joggers and racers—fast for many of the reputed benefits listed above. But they also have another reason to go without food. European research has proven that if a person "depletes" or uses up the sugar stored in the muscles for energy, then "reloads" the energy reserve by eating large quantities of carbohydrates, he or she initially will store twice the usual amount of sugar in the muscles. With twice as much fuel available, a runner can last longer and improve running performance. Many runners now prepare for races by depletion and reloading. Fasting, of course, will deplete the body's stored fuel quickly, because the body is no longer getting raw material to make into fuel. They usually fast for a few days until three days before the race, then begin eating a high-carbohydrate diet.

But the practice can be dangerous, warns Dr. George A. Sheehan, cardiologist, columnist, and author of a best-selling book, *Running and Being*. Individuals vary in their ability to replenish their fuel supply—some bodies take longer than others. An athlete running without fuel can get into trouble, and at the very least will end up feeling terrible. "Many try it and vow never to do it again," Sheehan says.

The reloading principle has proven effective, however. "But you don't have to fast to get the same results," Sheehan says. Sugar will be depleted after a high-protein, low-carbohydrate diet, too. If you follow that kind of diet until a few days before a race, then switch to a high-carbohydrate diet, you will also double the sugar reserve.

"Fasting," says Sheehan, "is a spiritual act, it has nothing to do with health." But running is a religious act, too, he adds, and that is where some runners make the connection between the two. "It has to do with lifestyle, not performance."

THE SENSATION OF FASTING

You have probably been tempted many times to ask what it actually feels like to fast. That is like asking what chocolate tastes like; it is difficult to make generalizations about it to someone who has never tried it.

But the persistence of fasting suggests that it is not unbearable, although for the first few days in particular it is not much fun. Generally, when the body is functioning properly, a faster goes through a few phases accompanied by different sensations. Although it takes some getting used to, the first day generally passes without much difficulty. You may get a hunger pang or two, but drinking water will dispel them. If you can get through the late-night snack period, you will probably sail through the night and next morning. On the second day, you keep sipping water but, by the dinner hour, you will get very hungry. Your stomach will continue to expect food, and muscle contractions will make it growl. Try not to watch television this second night; the food commercials can be killing.

That night, many people dream of food—hamburgers, roast beef, ice cream, things that really taste good to them. You may also get diarrhea or gas cramps. Some people get headaches. When you awake on the third day, you will still be hungry, but you will probably still feel energetic. Those feelings usually reverse sometime during the third or fourth day; your hunger will disappear, but you will begin to feel weak and perhaps tired and sleepy. Changes in your body, explained in chapter 8, should now keep you from getting really hungry until you have used up your stored energy in fat tissue. You will get bad breath and the coating on your tongue will appear. During this period, you may bounce back and forth between feeling weak and feeling energetic; this often depends on how much sleep you have been getting. From here on, experiences differ. Some people feel very peppy, others very weak. Much of what you experience probably depends on why you are fasting and what you believe about it.

7

the surest way to lose weight

BEING FAT is very much like being in prison. They both require a risky escape maneuver, good behavior, or a long term to win freedom. Even then, chances are very high that the "offender" will be back for another stretch. Most people who succeed at losing excess poundage regain most of the loss within five years.

Americans are quite familiar with this trapped feeling. What most of us eat no longer matches the lifestyle we lead of working at a desk, riding in cars and elevators, and sitting through our entertainment. Most of us have been touched by what doctors have dubbed the obesity epidemic; obesity is the major nutritional problem in the United States today. About forty thousand Americans are morbidly obese, that is, weighing more than 300 pounds or twice their ideal weight. Perhaps thirty-five million qualify as obese in medical parlance, which means they weigh more than 20 percent more than their optimum weight. The government estimates that a least seventy million Americans, including the two groups just mentioned, see a higher figure on the scale when they weigh themselves than they should. Other experts suggest that the total is even higher, perhaps half of the country's two-hundred-million-plus population. According to statistics from the National Center for Health Statistics, the average male carries around between 20 and 30 extra pounds, and the average female weighs between 15 and 30 pounds too many.

Like criminals, these people must pay for their "sin." They have a harder time making friends, buying clothes, even getting jobs or getting into college. Oral Roberts University last year began suspending students for being too fat and failing to lose weight in a given time period. A few years ago, a New York City-based employment agency conducted a survey of fifteen thousand executives and discovered that overweight bosses were earning less, for the same kind of jobs, than lean ones. The discrepancy averaged $1,000 in salary per pound. It also found that slim executives will get promoted more quickly. Psychological studies have concluded that attractive people, and a fat person is usually considered to be unattractive regardless of how lovely or handsome the face is, win over nonattractive people in many areas. Attractive people are assumed to be smarter, friendlier, sincerer, kinder, happier, more fun, and less likely to do wrong, regardless of realities.

Fat is dangerous to your health, most doctors and scientists agree. Heavies are more likely to get some forms of cancer, have heart trouble, and develop diseases such as diabetes, gout, degenerative arthritis, and gallbladder problems than their skinny counterparts. Excess flab can also aggravate existing diseases. Recently, following the flap about the carcinogenicity of the artificial sweetener saccharin, a physicist calculated that the risks of getting cancer from drinking saccharin-sweetened soft drinks are lower than the risk of health hazards produced by drinking sugared sodas and gaining weight.

It is no wonder, then, that over the last few decades, Americans have tried hundreds of different reducing diets and all kinds of tricks to shed extra weight. The Food and Drug Administration now estimates that about half the population goes on a reducing diet at least once a year. Other fatties probably consider reducing schemes, but cannot discipline themselves. A congressional study pegged the amount of money Americans spend on fad diets each year at $10 billion—and that does not include the vitamin supplements many take while they diet. Promoters have tried to hawk all kinds of gimmicks to help people stick to a diet, including powders to burn away fat, computers to keep track of food intake, and books galore.

Among the most recent is a novelty item meant as a joke—a

diet fork advertised as "a new twist in weight control." The silver-plated utensil, which sells for about seven dollars, sports curled tines that make picking up food impossible—in other words, a wink at fasting, one "risky maneuver" used to escape fat.

There is no doubt about it, fasting deserves its common billing as "the ultimate diet." If you want to shed pounds, there is no quicker, surer way to do it than by refraining from eating altogether. It is simple, with no complicated rules to follow and no addition to be completed. It is certainly the cheapest way to diet; there is no need to buy expensive protein foods or pills or appetite-suppressing candies required by other reducing regimens. And, although it looks as if it would be the most brutal diet, it is probably one of the easiest. Many dieters cannot stick to a low-calorie diet that requires abstention from all the good-tasting foods. They feel rather like Alice in her exchange with the Queen in Lewis Carroll's *Through the Looking Glass and What Alice Found There.*

> *"The rule is, jam tomorrow and jam yesterday—but never jam today."*
>
> *"It must come sometimes to 'jam today,'" Alice objected.*
>
> *"No, it can't," said the Queen. "It's jam every other day: today isn't any other day, you know."*

Few people, especially those who have trouble controlling their eating under normal conditions, can always be "good" in avoiding sweets and other fattening foods. But, with fasting, hunger usually disappears after the first two or three days; some people who cannot stay on reducing diets can suffer through a fast. Even Mahatma Gandhi recognized this. "Voluntary meagre eating is one of the most difficult things in the world," he wrote to Madeleine Slade in September 1933. "It is a perpetual fast much more difficult than the complete periodic fasts."

And fasting looks very effective, which makes it attractive to a dieter. Of course, the amount of weight lost will depend on the starting condition and weight of the faster, the prefast diet, the amount of activity during the fast, and other variables, but a faster can expect to lose between 1½ and 3¼ pounds during the first twenty-four hours. It could take two weeks on some diets to lose the same amount. If you continue fasting, you will probably continue to shed pounds rapidly—about 2 pounds each day if you are very overweight—on each of the next ten days. From then on, the loss diminishes gradually until toward the end of the second month of a fast you will be losing a little more than ½ pound a day. That pace then remains fairly constant.

Despite this effectiveness, most doctors continue to disapprove of fasting unless the risks of chronic obesity are more hazardous to health than the risks associated with fasting. If you have only 10 or 15 or even 25 pounds to lose, most doctors would say you do not qualify. However, many people in this category are successfully fasting to turn svelte. As one woman at a fasting farm, where the undisciplined can stop eating with no temptations to lure them off the fast, said, "Everybody's getting the idea because they have tried everything else and nothing works. There is a lot of pressure to be thin."

Over the centuries, some doctors have prescribed fasting as treatment for obesity. Europeans use it more frequently than Americans. Scientific research on it goes back at least as far as 1915, but it was not considered in earnest by most doctors until the 1950s. Then, in 1959, a British doctor advocated fasting for obese patients. In the United States, Dr. Garfield Duncan assumed a pioneering role. During the late 1950s, Duncan took obese patients who turned to fasting as a last resort into his care. He admitted heavyweights who had already tried everything else to lose weight to a Philadelphia hospital. They began ten- or twelve-day supervised fasts on which they drank only water, coffee, and tea. Duncan and his assistants gave them a multivitamin pill, weighed them, and took blood and urine samples to test every day. The patients also were instructed in what they should eat when they went home—daily diets totaling 900 to 1,500 calories. Patients could, if they regained weight very quickly or if they needed to see faster weight loss, fast at home, unsupervised, for a day or two at a time. If necessary, they could also return every few months for another long fast at the hospital.

Duncan's patients got adequate, but not spectacular, results for their troubles. After fourteen months of dieting, including four twelve-day fasts broken by periods of calorie-watching at home, one typical patient dropped from 303 pounds to 217 pounds. Another, after twenty-seven months of dieting that entailed four fasts at the hospital, a few two-day fasts at home, and plenty of willpower in between, shed 93 pounds. He ended the diet weighing 272 pounds.

By comparison, if these people had been able to stick to a diet with 800 calories fewer each day than the body needed for fuel, the first patient would have lost about the same amount—84 pounds instead of the actual 86-pound loss. But the second patient would have lost as much as 162 pounds, according to medical researchers' calculations.

What is more, the slow, deliberate weight loss may have been easier to maintain. Duncan's patients did fairly well in this area, but not as well as would be expected if the patients followed the calorie-watching program. After two years, thirty-seven of Duncan's fifty-seven patients had maintained their weight loss or lost even more. Ten had gained back some weight, and ten regained all or more than they had lost. Other fasters have not done even that well. In several experiments, researchers discovered that although obese patients can take off hefty amounts of weight over a month's time—usually between 25 and 65 pounds—they regain it. Most slip back into old habits of overeating. They found that within less than a year's time, all the good accomplished by the fast is undone.

So some researchers decided to keep obese patients on longer fasts, making them lose more weight, on the theory that they would then be less likely to regain it all. If people are closer to their ideal weight, they look good—they may feel so pleased about being slimmer that they will watch what they eat more closely.

But this approach did not bring the desired results either, for three main reasons.

As in any diet, at first the weight comes off very quickly, but later the losses are less dramatic. For people who are eating nothing, this can be very discouraging. If they cannot lose more weight by starving themselves, they think, how can they lose weight? Why should a person eating nothing but using energy experience the same plateaus a calorie-counting dieter does? For one thing, as a person continues on a fast, the body goes through several changes, one of them being a slowdown in body metabolism. Fasters sometimes feel weak and may cut back their activity without realizing it. But even if they did not, the less food one eats, the less energy the body uses up—involuntarily. On any constant reducing diet, the rate of loss will decrease over time, regardless of the person's activity level. (Conversely, whenever a person eats, the metabolism rate goes up. That is one reason why overweight people in particular should eat breakfast; it gets the body moving at a faster rate early in the day.) Doctors do not yet understand why this happens; new methods of measuring energy expenditure have only recently confirmed this theory. It may have something to do with hormones, some theorize. As if that were not enough, the body endures another change during a fast that slows weight loss. Initially, the body manufactures most of its needed fuel from lean tissue. As time passes, however, more and more fat is consumed and turned into fuel. Both of these processes, which are explained in the next chapter, are the reverse of the way the body digests food. Fat contains more energy per gram than either protein or carbohydrate (one reason why most diets ask for a big reduction in fat intake). Scientists have calculated that 1 gram of fat contains the energy equivalent of 9 calories, while 1 gram of protein or carbohydrate can only provide about 4 calories. Therefore, in fasting, when you dissolve 1 gram of fat to provide fuel, you are getting more energy than 1 gram of lean tissue supplies.

Second, once a faster quits that regimen and begins a period of refeeding, there is no way to escape regaining some of the weight lost. That will happen no matter what the dieter eats. Why? During any quick drop in weight, most of the loss can be attributed to a loss in water from body tissues. This is true to some extent on almost any diet and even more so on a crash diet. When the body is not getting enough energy from food, it draws on its reserves of glycogen (a starchy carbohydrate) for fuel. But glycogen, stored in the liver and in the muscles, is combined with water. As it is used, the water is no longer needed, so the body eliminates it. A faster also uses a good deal of lean tissue to make fuel, more than individuals on a balanced reducing diet. Lean tissue contains plenty of water, sodium, and other minerals that regulate the retention of this water. As lean tissue is mobilized for fuel, the minerals are no longer needed, and the water they hold also runs out of the body. Researchers estimate that for every pound of lean tissue the body uses to make fuel, you will lose 4 pounds of water weight. As soon as you resume eating, the body replaces the lean tissue it used up—and it therefore will add more water to its weight. And as soon as you eat anything with salt or another form of sodium, water will be retained again. These swings in weight loss, when the food consumed could not possibly account for the gain, are disheartening, to say the least. They are often enough to spur more eating, and more weight is regained.

Third, despite the big losses in poundage, many fasters continue to look fat, puffy, and unattractive. This occurs because the quality of weight loss is not as good as it is on a longer, slower diet that results in the same number of pounds lost. Slower weight losses result in a bigger decrease in fat cells. For example, one group of researchers put seven obese women on fasts ranging from ten to forty-five weeks. They lost between 54 and 146 pounds. But by measuring various decreases in nitrogen and putting the fasters through other tests, the researchers calculated that only half the weight drop was a loss of fat tissue (thus a damaging amount of lean tissue is lost even on prolonged fasts, even though the longer a fast lasts, the lower the proportion of lean tissue lost). Two of these women showed no change whatsoever in the proportion of body fat after losing all those pounds. In another experiment, researchers used the same group of subjects on two occasions to test the fat lost during different diets. On a total fast, almost 65 percent of the weight change was due to a loss of lean tissue, while the remaining 35 percent represented fat loss. In contrast, on a low-calorie, high-fat diet, the dieters lost only 3 percent of the drop in lean tissue. On a sixteen-day experiment in fasting, researchers calculated that only 15 percent of the weight loss was fat tissue. Thus the idea of a long fast making a patient lose so much weight that he or she would try harder to keep it off did not work; the big loss did not make the patients look better until and unless they maintained the loss long enough for the body to lose more fat.

Because the quality of weight reduction is poor, the maintenance success rate usually low, and the destruction of body protein so great, most doctors continue to frown on prolonged fasting as a weight-reducing diet except for some extremely obese persons. In some cases, fasting for a long period of time has caused death. The story of one Englishwoman, mentioned already in chapter 1, is legendary. She had lost more than half her lean body tissue; several organs—including her heart—had atrophied. In another case, a nineteen-year-old girl died after thirty-three weeks of fasting. But, in all, medical literature records only about twenty deaths resulting from total fasting. These are not insignificant, but neither should they be used as scare tactics. To repeat, no one should go on a fast of more than a few days without consulting a doctor and without supervision. Most doctors will even insist on hospitalization if the fast is to last longer than ten days. But controlled fasting can be used as a diet, in its proper place. Generally, some doctors will accept fasting of up to two weeks for very obese patients. Others can fast intermittently with better results anyhow. Researchers have discovered that short, intermittent fasts can result in a weight loss of which 80 percent will be from burning fat tissue.

Besides the associated dangers, the medical world faults fasting as a weight reducer because it does not attack the root of the problem; it does not change behavior to allow the overeater to cope with temptation once the fast is over. Some doctors compare fasting, as well as other dieting techniques, to the pill in a story of a person who is having trouble getting to sleep every night because his neighbors are chronically noisy. He takes a sleeping pill, which may help him get to sleep, but it does not solve the problem. Sooner or later, the pill will lose its effectiveness, and the person still cannot sleep. (Indeed, fasting is less effective the second time around.) Obesity is a misunderstood environmental problem that is not a matter of weakness of character; even many doctors have not gotten this word from their researcher colleagues. Dieters must revamp their eating and activity habits to effect a permanent weight loss. Feelings about food must also be thought out; guilt has been associated with eating ever since Eve ate the wrong apple in the Garden of Eden. That and other emotions and attitudes about food must be reworked. Fasting can help do that.

Actually, the best use of fasting among the nonobese who may be just a little pudgy is probably as a weight-maintenance device. Medical experts agree that keeping weight off is much harder for those prone to be overweight that losing it in the first place. Many people—including model Cheryl Tiegs and actor Van Johnson—reportedly fast on Mondays after a food-filled weekend to maintain their correct weight. Fasting can also be useful as a first step in a longer calorie-counting diet. It will give the psychological lift of taking off the first few pounds very quickly. Even though 1 or 2 pounds will be regained, if the faster understands what is happening, that little weight increment does not have to be demoralizing.

One woman has another novel approach to dieting that uses

fasting—sort of. "I tell myself all day long that I am going to fast. I usually cannot make it through the entire day, but I don't start eating until it becomes unbearable—and I cut out a lot of food that I otherwise would have eaten had I begun eating with breakfast," she says. Hers is hardly a regimen doctors would recommend (they remind us that eating food so close to bedtime adds pounds because the body's metabolism slows during sleep), but it works for her. And who can knock that?

MODIFIED FASTS

When all nourishment for the body is curtailed, that is a total fast—whether it lasts one day or twenty-five days or ten months. Anything else that people call fasting is really a modified fast. Doctors usually call these regimens "semistarvation," meaning that nutrient intake is dramatically lowered. Reducing calorie intake from more than 2,000 calories a day, which is about the lowest amount an average-sized adult would consume, to say 400 calories a day would definitely qualify. Many dieters attack their weight problem with that kind of "fast."

Among health-conscious modified fasters, juice fasts win much praise. These fasters supplement their sipping of pure water with varying amounts of orange, lemon, tomato, carrot, grapefruit, and many other kinds of fruit and vegetable juices. Sometimes the juices are used at full strength, but many times fasters dilute them with water. Other fasters drink cups of hot beef or chicken bouillon or clear vegetable broth. Every now and then you may find a modified fasting advocate who will also eat celery, cabbage, a carrot or two, or another very low-calorie vegetable on occasion. But the problem with these diets is the same as it is with all low-calorie routines—the dieter gets hungry. Unless the dieter has unbendable will power, the diet cannot last very long. As already mentioned, hunger disappears on a total fast. But juice, soup, and vegetables all contain carbohydrates, and carbohydrates trigger the secretion of the hormone insulin. Insulin stimulates the brain's hunger center, telling it to crave food. Under that pressure, the fast is often broken before the faster intended to resume eating a normal diet.

Recognizing the clinical benefits of fasting in obesity, medical researchers for years have kept busy searching for a way to adapt fasting so that it would be less dangerous but almost as effective. Finding a routine that did not stir up hunger but also did not use up large amounts of lean body tissue to make body fuel would keep the benefits but eliminate the drawbacks of total fasting. For a long time, they tried the same approach as juice fasters. They experimented with feeding a dieter small amounts of carbohydrates, the raw material for the body's principal source of energy during normal times—glucose. Researchers thought they could design a diet with just the right amount and kind of carbohydrates to keep the brain in fuel, to let the rest of the body adapt to using fat tissue as raw material for additional fuel needed by the rest of the body, and to prevent the destruction of lean body tissue. But it did not work—they could not keep the dieter from getting hungry. Carbohydrates always stimulate hunger.

It takes a long involved process, but fat tissue can be broken down and rebuilt into glucose, too. But not as easily as protein tissue can—that is why the body first uses lean tissue to produce fuel during a total fast. What would happen if dieters ate just enough protein to be transformed into glucose for the brain? It could impede the destruction of lean tissue, and yet it does not provoke hunger. Researchers searched for a routine that would provide just enough protein to satisfy the brain's need for glucose, preserve lean body tissues, and yet allow the body to burn up fat tissue for the rest of its necessary energy. Dr. George L. Blackburn, an associate professor at Harvard Medical School, did it. He developed a "protein-sparing fast," as the medical world tagged the regimen, which initially called for 4 to 12 ounces of solid protein—in the form of lean meat, fish, or poultry—each day. The first test cases also took vitamin and mineral supplements. It worked—patients lost weight. In two projects with a total of 167 patients, 81 percent lost weight according to projections. After a year, half of them had lost 40 pounds, and two-thirds of them maintained the loss for at least a year after the fast. Less than a third kept it all off for two years, but at least the idea was working.

Using Blackburn's idea as inspiration, other medical researchers began experimenting with protein-sparing fasts—with good results. A team in Cleveland, headed by Dr. Sol Genuth, treated about twelve hundred very obese patients over a four-year period. One person lost 300 pounds, and had maintained the loss when the fourth anniversary of the fast's end passed. Other losses ranged from 35 pounds to 124 pounds, with a decrease of 78 pounds as the mean. On the average, men lost 4½ pounds a week, while women lost 3 pounds.

Follow-up studies showed that after two years, about 50 percent of the total amount lost by the entire group had been regained. Some individuals did well, however: almost one-tenth did not put a single pound back on.

Promoters soon picked up the diet and sold it to an estimated two to four million people in 1977. "Predigested liquid protein" became a familiar sight on drugstore shelves, even though it sold for at least fifteen dollars a quart. For that price, dieters get to choke down 6 to 8 ounces of this liquid each day. The elixir is actually a gelatin material made by boiling down cattle and hog hides and tendons and adding sweeteners, colorings, flavorings, preservatives, and sometimes minerals and vitamins. The dieter must also swallow a megavitamin capsule, folic acid tablets, and a potassium supplement each day. By so doing, he or she can expect to shed perhaps 7 to 15 pounds the first week and 25 pounds in the first month. Promoters say that about 80 percent of those who try the diet stick with it long enough to lose what they set out to jettison.

But there are dangers associated with the liquid protein diet fad. Some people on it died. Medical authorities pin some of the blame on the diet, which they say contributed to the deaths of at least sixteen persons. Many more cases of death and illness are still being studied to determine the cause of death. Those who died had lost a great deal of weight, often between 30 and 40 percent of total body weight at the start of the diet. Of the first ten cases, for example, each had lost an average of 90 pounds and had followed the diet for several weeks or months. Most of the sixteen deaths occurred after the patient's heart began beating irregularly. Doctors are still studying the connection between the diet and the deaths, and there is still no definitive word, but they suggest a few possible theories: perhaps, for example, because the body gives up potassium, which carries some of the body's electrical signals, normal electrical impulses in the heart are short-circuited. Others suggest that liquid protein may contain an unknown harmful substance that exerts itself only after several weeks or months of use. Some researchers have proposed that the long period without food results in the deficit of some crucial element—as yet undiscovered—other than potassium.

Even promoters warn that the liquid protein diet should only be used by obese people, but many relatively thin people began to try it, at least at first. Doctors grew more and more alarmed when more and more people began administering the diet themselves, without the benefit of a recent physical examination, blood and urine tests, and knowledge of what physical conditions would preclude its use. Persons with heart, liver, or kidney trouble, or with a tendency toward those diseases, should not diet this way, but seeing a doctor can be expensive. Many who set up clinics to supervise liquid protein diets charged as much as $150 for the first visit and $60 a week thereafter. Doctors expressed concern about the false sense of security the diet creates; people think they are getting all vital bodily needs, and they carry on normal activity without realizing that the body is subject to additional stress. Some brands of liquid protein on the market are not of the highest quality; many do not contain minerals needed as electrical conductors. The Food and Drug Administration even recalled a few shipments of the product. Last year the FDA moved to require manufacturers of liquid protein to print a warning label on each package explaining that such a low-calorie diet may cause illness or death and should always be used under medical supervision. The FDA also sponsored some research on rats. After less than a month of being fed only liquid protein, 95 percent of two hundred rats had died—mostly from irregular heartbeats, just like most of the human deaths. Researchers warned against making a judgment based on this preliminary information but, nevertheless, they cautioned dieters to consume the prescribed amount of liquid protein; many people were skimping to cause a higher weight loss, but the tests showed that rats fed the least amount of it died earliest.

The frightening part about these human deaths is that many of them occurred among people who were being supervised by doctors. In other words, difficulties could not be predicted by medical tests or examinations. So although the liquid protein diet at first showed promise of being the biggest advance in weight control in years, most doctors are leery of it. Many are waiting until more research is done and more questions are answered before giving approval. Even Blackburn, the originator of the concept, reportedly still has many reservations about its use.

The diet also comes in for criticism because it—like total fasting—does not attack the environmental and behavioral roots of overweight. But many weight specialists hope the problems with protein-sparing fasts can be worked out soon. Genuth, for example, has had four deaths in his program—one of normal causes and three in patients with prior evidence of heart disease. He admits the dangers involved and is particularly concerned that the long-term effects of this kind of diet are unknown; his own program, one of the first, is only seven years old. But Genuth feels the approach is worthwhile because it works and because dieters will stick with it. It brings dieters down to a weight from which they can be taught how to change their eating and living habits. "If I could get patients to stick to a one thousand calorie a day diet, I would use it," he says. "But they won't do it."

The diet also wins points because it can be done on an outpatient basis, unlike a total fast, which most doctors feel should be conducted at a hospital.

8

how the body adjusts to a fast

An obese, middle-aged woman in Scotland once took no food for two hundred fifty-nine days, lost 74 pounds, and lived to tell about it, the story goes. But what happened to her body during those eight months? More important, what happens to the body of someone who fasts for two weeks a couple of times a year? And what will happen to your body if you skip every meal for several days?

Before you fast, you should know exactly what is going on inside your body during the period it is not getting nourishment. The human body is remarkably adaptable and resilient; it often takes care of ills by itself. When it does need help, we usually just turn the whole problem over to a doctor. Consequently, we are often ill-informed about the way our own body works. This is changing. We are beginning to understand that many decisions we make daily affect our health, and that to make those decisions we need background information. Just to see if you are ready to fast, answer the true-or-false questions in the following quiz. If you can answer them all correctly (see the end of the chapter), you are ready to make the decision.

1. It is essential for a faster to drink large quantities of water. After several weeks without food, he or she must drink at least 2 quarts of water each day.
2. Glucose, a simple sugar, is the body's main energy source. On a long fast, the liver manufactures the normal amount of glucose required, drawing on fat and muscle tissue, until the faster eats again.
3. The longer you fast, the higher the rate of lean tissue loss.
4. You're doing a little ironing as you watch television. At this moment, your brain is consuming most of the energy your body can provide.
5. The body keeps its most readily usable store of reserve fuel in the form of glycogen, which can be converted back into glucose by the liver. The average adult warehouses the equivalent of about 760 calories of glycogen, which is about the same number contained in a 4-ounce piece of T-bone steak and a small dish of chocolate ice cream.
6. In fact, the storehouse of glycogen in the liver usually is not big enough to last for the duration of the period between dinner and breakfast.
7. If you eat a heavy meal, it will be digested as usual and converted into amino acids and glucose (sugar). The blood will then carry much more sugar as it circulates through the body.
8. Just as on any reducing diet, hunger pangs will come and go frequently throughout a ten-day fast.

That's it—not an easy test. It points out that what the body does during a fast is not simple. You could ask your doctor to supply the answers. If you plan to stop eating for more than a day or two, you should see your doctor for a physical examination and an explanation. But most doctors are dead set against fasting, for any reason. They may play up the effects in negative terms, referring to excessive protein breakdown, mineral imbalances, and withering away of lean muscle tissue. Other physicians may be more willing to tell the whole story, but demands on their time often require them to give a quick analysis in a mix of medical mumbo jumbo: "catabolism," "negative energy balance," "autolysis," and so on. So the answers to the quiz are sprinkled throughout the explanation that follows, with a reference back to the question number. For those of you who must know the answers now, they are also listed at the end of the chapter. But even if you understand the physiological aspects of fasting, you must still see a doctor before you fast and during it if you intend to undertake a prolonged fast.

THE BASIC FACTS

To survive, the human body needs water and a good mix of proteins, carbohydrates, and fats. If the diet is as varied as it should be, natural food will supply the necessary vitamins and minerals. Carbohydrates provide an immediate source of energy for the body. They are turned into glucose, which can be used on the spot as you go through daily functions and activities such as swimming, skiing, doing housework, playing tennis and running to catch the bus. Fruit, sugar, honey, oatmeal, rice, and peas are all carbohydrates. Proteins—chicken, fish, eggs, and lean red meats, for example—take part in the bodily functions called metabolism, the chemical changes that are the result of body tissue activity. When digested, proteins break down into the basic, essential material that makes up living cells. They are necessary for tissue synthesis, that is, for the building, maintaining, and repairing of the heart, skin, brain, lungs, nerve system, skeletal muscle, nails, and hair. Protein can also supply energy. Fats provide energy, too, usually after carbohydrates have been used up. They also carry some vitamins, keep the skin from drying out, and make up the tissue that insulates the body. This fat tissue, however, is basically inactive; it usually does not contribute to metabolism.

Unfortunately, Americans in general eat the wrong mix of foods. Government statistics indicate that the average person's diet consists of about 12 percent protein, 22 percent complex carbohyrate such as fruits and vegetables, 24 percent sugar, and 42 percent fats. Although nutritionists disagree on what amounts would be "most healthful," they do agree that only the percentage of protein consumed is about right. Fat should be lowered to about 30 percent and sugar to about 15 percent. The remaining 21 percent should be added to the complex carbohydrate category, for a total of 43 percent.

If we eat a healthy diet, about 70 percent of the body, by weight, is water. About 20 percent is protein, the chief constituent of the body's soft tissue. The rest is mostly fat.

The body's active, living tissue is constantly being renewed. Old tissue breaks down in a process called catabolism, and new cells are formed to replace them in a process called anabolism. Scientists estimate that about one-third to one-half of the body's protein—the essential material in cells—is in this state of flux on any normal day. But the body does not keep a reserve supply of protein for this renewal. It must come from the protein we eat. Before it can be used by the body, the protein must go through the digestive process to be broken down into amino acids. These amino acids contain many elements, including carbon, hydrogen, oxygen, usually sulfur, and occasionally iron and phosphorus. The key component of protein, however, is nitrogen; it makes up about 16 percent of a protein molecule. Researchers measure the amount of nitrogen excreted by the body in urine to determine how much protein the body is losing during a fast.

We have already said that the body needs fuel—glucose—to perform these vital metabolic functions. It also converts food into usable energy through digestion. Like the proteins that break down into amino acids, carbohydrates and fats also go through radical structural changes as they travel through the digestive system. The food is constantly being broken down from larger molecules to smaller ones that can be absorbed by the body. Carbohydrates eventually become glucose, and fats convert to fatty acids and glycerol. This boiling-down process begins in the mouth and continues in the stomach, where gastric juices go to work on pieces of food. Some fluids that are ready to be absorbed by the body leave the stomach through its walls. The rest of the food passes into the small intestine, a 30-foot tube where enzymes and bile continue to break it down. The digestible portion then slips through the small intestine's walls for use, while the remainder proceeds through the large intestine to be eliminated by the body.

Blood carries around the nutrients that are the end products of digestion. But before it circulates through the body, blood that has been enriched by digested food first goes to the liver. The liver filters out impurities and toxins. But it also performs another important function: it removes excess glucose, keeping the sugar level of the blood fairly constant at all times. The liver recombines this excess glucose into a carbohydrate called glycogen that it can store for use when the body is not getting enough energy. This wouldn't be necessary if we all ate the exact amount of food we needed each day for energy but, of course, we do not. (Therefore the answer to question 7 in the quiz at the beginning of this chapter is false. Even if you eat a heavy meal, the body continues to get a steady supply of sugar.)

These processes happen every day as the normal way the body uses food to provide power for its activities and to make tissue. They are also the processes that must adapt when we stop eating. The body cannot slip into an "off" position. Even when a person sleeps, a minimal level of activity continues. He or she must still get energy for life to continue. Each individual's needs differ according to activity level, body size, body makeup (remember that fat tissue is basically inactive and does not need to be supplied with energy, although the body needs fuel to carry it around), environment, and various other factors. But nutritionists suggest that moderately active people need an average of about 15 calories per pound of body weight each day to maintain (neither gain nor lose) weight. A 120-pound woman, therefore, should be eating about 1,800 calories a day, while a 160-pound man can eat about 2,400 calories a day. The latest statistics from the U.S. Department of Commerce, however, indicate that Americans are eating much more than that, which is why we have so many problems with obesity. In 1976, the average daily caloric intake was more than 3,100 calories per person.

Researchers have also calculated the body's need for protein, since needed amino acids to build new body cells must come from protein foods. The National Academy of Sciences recommends that people eat about 65 grams—which is a little more than 2 ounces—of protein each day. Actually, that is about twice what the body needs each day to replace protein lost, but the excess is merely transformed into glucose for fuel or stored as fat.

HOW THE BODY ADAPTS

When outside nourishment stops, the human body first begins to draw needed energy from the glucose reserve the liver stored away as glycogen. The brain now throws the storage mechanism into reverse. Blood passing by the small intestine enters the liver with a lower than normal concentration of glucose. It picks up some of the stored glycogen, which the liver has converted back to glucose, before circulating throughout the body.

The brain uses more glucose than any other part of the body. When you are at rest, scientists have estimated, your brain consumes about two-thirds of the glucose produced by the body. (Therefore the answer to question 4 is true.) If the blood's sugar level drops rapidly, the brain has trouble functioning; the person sometimes becomes confused or exhibits erratic behavior. If the sugar deficiency lasts long enough, the person can lapse into a coma and even die. So the body acts to keep the brain steadily supplied with glucose.

Generally, it takes 100 to 150 grams of glucose[1] to satisfy the brain and nervous system's demand for energy each day. That equals 400 to 600 calories of carbohydrates or proteins. The remaining amount of required glucose, which is between 50 and 75 grams or 200 to 300 calories, goes mainly to supply energy to red blood cells and to muscles attached to the skeleton. These figures, however, apply only when the body is at rest. When a person steps up activity, the body's demand for glucose goes up, too.

George F. Cahill, Jr., a doctor associated with Harvard University (and who, incidentally, was one of those who first suggested that the high-protein, ketogenic diet, later popularized in books by Dr. Stillman and Dr. Atkins, would take off more pounds than normal, varied diets with the same number of calories), has measured the energy stores of normal and obese adults.[2] Cahill found that any adult, trim or obese, stores only the equivalent of 280 calories of glycogen in the liver. That amount, in the form of glucose, weighs only about 100 grams. With a brain demand of 100 to 150 grams of glucose each day and a reservoir in the liver of only 100 grams, the brain could be left without fuel in a matter of hours.

What is more, some of the liver's cache of glycogen is kept as a more or less emergency stockpile, and ordinarily it will not be given up by the liver immediately. So even less time elapses

[1] Vernon R. Young and Nevin S. Scrimshaw, "The Physiology of Starvation," *Scientific American* 225 (October 1971):16.

[2] Quoted in *Scientific American* (October 1971):16.

before the liver's available store of glycogen ordinarily is exhausted. "In fact," say Vernon R. Young and Nevin S. Scrimshaw in an article published by *Scientific American* in October 1971, "the stored glucose is not sufficient for the duration of the overnight fast between dinner and breakfast." (Therefore, the answer to question 6 is false.)

The body does keep another reserve of glycogen. Cahill discovered that an adult of normal weight stored glycogen equivalent to about 480 calories in muscle tissue. In an obese person, this amount increases to about 640 calories. (The answer to question 5 is true; add the calorie equivalents of glycogen stored in the liver and stored in muscle.)

Fat tissue is the body's most important stockpile of energy. It can supply enormous amounts—equivalent to 141,000 calories in a normal adult and 752,000 calories in an obese adult, Cahill says. Unfortunately, the body cannot transform this fat into glucose very readily. So it must turn to the lean tissue, the protein tissue, which Cahill says stores the equivalent of 24,000 calories in a normal adult and 32,000 calories in an obese one. As soon as the body uses up all the stored glycogen, it begins to manufacture glucose from lean tissue through a process called gluconeogenesis.

The body transforms tissue into fuel in exactly the reverse way the tissue was formed from nutrients in the first place. Ordinarily, only old and unhealthy tissue dissolves into its components—amino acids, water, carbon dioxide, fatty acids, and so on—in a process called autolysis. But now the body converts healthy tissue into molecules that can be regrouped to provide the needed energy. Just as enzymes accomplished the breakdown of food in digestion, enzymes also break down the body's tissue. Scientists have detected and measured the presence of amino acids in the blood only a few hours after a meal has been digested, but after it would have been absorbed. That, they say, indicates how quickly the body draws raw materials from skeletal muscles for synthesis by the liver of glucose needed by the brain and nervous system. Other parts of the body, meanwhile, make use of the free fatty acids, given up by fat tissue, for energy.

As this process takes place, during the first few days of fasting, the cells are melting into their components, and that includes minerals, which the body eliminates. Sodium, potassium, calcium, magnesium, and other minerals are lost sometimes causing side effects, even severe ones. Low potassium levels, for example, can cause heart problems. "The mineral deficits are the single greatest potential hazard in a fast longer than two weeks," says Dr. Robert G. Campbell, who is associated with the University of Rochester Medical School. In some states, minerals are available at a drugstore without a prescription. But Campbell warns that taking mineral supplements without knowing whether or not they are actually needed can be more harmful than going without them.

With the mineral loss goes a large amount of water, which is the reason for most of a faster's early weight loss. The drop in pounds will vary, but a very obese person can lose as much as 8 pounds in the first twenty-four hours. More trim people will probably lose between 1½ and 3 pounds during the first day, then continue to lose an average of 2 pounds each day for the next several.

For a while after you stop eating, your stomach will continue to secrete gastric juices, as it usually does. It may also go through the normal muscular contractions of the digestive process. Some people experience these as hunger pangs. Generally, if you drink a glass of water, the hunger will go away. Your body needs some water to prevent it from becoming dehydrated and to prevent damage to the kidneys. Take water as you need it and want it, but there is no need to force it down. Water can also supply some minerals. Some fasting advocates recommend drinking at least 2 quarts of water each day. But in fasts of more than a few days, the body has its own protective system that conserves water. One medical study determined that if a faster is not sweating excessively, a cup of water each day is enough to maintain the body's water balance. (Therefore, the answer to question 1 is false.)

DURING A LONG FAST

If you are only going to fast for a few days, you can stop reading about what happens to your body right here. Only normal, everyday body processes have taken place, but catabolism—the breaking down of tissue—has occurred at a much higher rate than usual. During this initial period, protein from lean tissue provides most of the raw materials for the manufacture of fuel. The basic rate of body metabolism drops, however, which conserves some of the protein that might otherwise be lost. It can decrease by 20 to 25 percent as the pulse rate slows, the blood pressure drops, and so forth. Still, a significant amount of protein is metabolized for energy. Take, for example, the liver. "In dietary protein deficiency the liver loses twenty to thirty percent of its total protein content within a few days," according to *Modern Nutrition in Health and Disease*, the medical bible of nutrition. (Fortunately, the liver is usually a regenerative organ and can restore itself to health if proper nourishment resumes.)

Researchers can gauge the amount of protein lost by measuring the amount of nitrogen eliminated by the body in urine, but they do not know how much body protein can be consumed without interfering drastically with bodily functions. In one case in which a faster died, doctors discovered that the woman had lost about half the lean tissue in her body. Her heart had been severely damaged. This woman, however, had fasted for 210 days. Her weight dropped from 260 pounds to 132 pounds. She died nine days after she went off the fast.

That was an extreme case, however, and one of the few supervised fasts recorded in medical literature that ended tragically. Although protein loss continues for the duration of any fast, the rate of loss is highest at the beginning of a fast. (Therefore, the answer to question 3 is false.) If the original pace continued during the entire fast, a person could not survive for very long. Some doctors estimate that three weeks would be the longest a human could hang on if the body did not adapt. Tissues other than the brain and nervous system have long since begun to use the products of fat tissue breakdown for fuel and, after the first few days that a person goes without food, the brain does, too. It continues to demand the same or nearly the same energy equivalent. But now it switches its main source of fuel to one the body can more readily produce. Catabolism of fat tissue can still produce about 16 grams of glucose each day, and lean tissue breakdown now supplies about 8 grams of glucose each day. For the rest of its needed energy, the brain begins to utilize substances called ketone bodies, or keto acids. They can be produced by the breakdown of fatty tissue more easily than glucose because they are intermediate products of the catabolic process. Making ketone bodies from fat does not require all of the steps that making glucose does. (The answer to question 2 is false.) You can compare it to making a potato dish: you can serve boiled potatoes, but they are also an intermediate step in making mashed potatoes.

The body begins making ketone bodies about the third day of a fast, but the concentration of them in the bloodstream must rise to a high level before the brain starts utilizing them for fuel. Researchers have found that the mobilization of body protein for energy—through the process of gluconeogenesis—drops off on about the seventh day of fasting. That, apparently, is when the brain has settled in to using ketones as its primary fuel.

When the brain does switch from using glucose as its main fuel to using ketones, a condition known as ketosis results. Ketosis is just a term for a high level of ketone bodies in the blood; it also occurs when you eat high-protein, low-carbohydrate diets. The presence of ketones in the blood sometimes acts as an appetite suppressant, helping to keep a dieter on the diet or fast. (Therefore, the answer to question 8 is false.) But ketosis also has side effects. Symptoms vary, but a person can become nauseated, dizzy, listless, tired, or irritable.

For most people in good health, however, these side effects of ketosis are not serious. And doctors find that the heavily overweight (in particular) can lose much more weight on a ketogenic diet than they can on a regular, low-calorie regimen. That is why doctors are willing to put patients on low-carbohydrate ketogenic diets; the health dangers associated with obesity can be much more dangerous than the side effects of ketosis.

The medical world still does not understand exactly how the brain can substitute ketone bodies for glucose as its fuel. Nor has it figured out a way to induce ketosis artificially, perhaps at an earlier stage in a reducing diet or fast. Some believe that two hormones secreted by the pancreas may have a role in the exchange. In normal times, insulin and glucagon keep glucose production in balance. Insulin stimulates conversion of glucose to glycogen for storage in the liver; glucagon encourages transformation from glygogen to glucose, for use as fuel. In other words, insulin stimulates the synthesis of fat, while glucagon enhances the breakdown of fat tissue. During fasting, researchers have found, naturally, that the insulin level of the body decreases and the glucagon level increases. Perhaps the different balance of these two hormones also influences the way the body utilizes the products of fat and protein tissues during a fast.

As a fast continues, the body goes through several changes: you may lose more hair than usual, your skin may feel drier, and you may get muscle cramps. Some people have diarrhea at the start of a fast. You may feel more sensitive to cold. You may feel tired and irritable. You may feel dizzy, because of blood pressure changes. Some people even experience changes in personality, although this generally occurs only on long fasts; it sometimes has to do with the change in perception of your body. We have already mentioned that your metabolism rate has dropped, so you may feel sluggish. Your pulse rate can decrease by five to ten beats per minute.

But these are minor side effects. Doctors who oppose fasting worry about more serious consequences that can also result. If you do not drink enough liquids, you can damage your kidneys, a possibility on all ketogenic diets. The increase in blood acidity caused by ketosis can also impair kidney function, increasing the retention of uric acid and possibly provoking a gout attack in someone who has gout. It can also give rise to gout in a person who previously had only a tendency toward the disease, which is marked by painful inflammation of joints. Doctors say the most serious side effect, however, can be caused by the higher level of fats in the blood. That is a dangerous condition for people with heart trouble or latent heart disease. Fasting can also bring on nervous tremors and cause severe headaches. Women may stop menstruating.

Tolerance for fasting and the ability to survive a fast depend on many individual factors, including the original state of health, body weight, body fat, temperature, humidity levels, amount of physical activity, and general environmental conditions. Many of these factors influence one another—another good reason to see a doctor if you intend to fast.

But you should also listen to your body; it can give you its own warnings. If you fast for several days and hunger has disappeared because you are in a ketotic state, watch for the return of hunger. Ketosis stops when you start eating carbohydrates again, however, so if you stop and start fasts intermittently, you will probably experience hunger throughout the period—or at least more often than if you stayed on a total fast. But if you have not broken a long fast, start eating again when hunger returns. Hunger signals that the body has given up most of its fat reserves. Its return warns that unless food is consumed again, the body will have to start cannibalizing essential lean tissues. Except this time there will be no mechanism to stop the high rate of protein breakdown once it has begun. The body would have no place to turn for another fuel.

Quiz answers

1. False; 2. False; 3. False; 4. True; 5. True; 6. True; 7. False; 8. False.

9
how to fast

LOU ZIEGLER IS a typical American: he read the directions but he did not really follow them. At twenty-eight, Ziegler enjoyed good health but, by his own admission, was more than slightly chubby. He decided to reduce by fasting. But his carelessness with the rules landed him in a hospital emergency room. It was nothing serious, mind you, but it gave him plenty of discomfort.

In the summer of 1977, Ziegler tipped the scales at about 200 pounds, 35 too many for a man with his height and build. The reporter for a Rochester, New York, newspaper had already shed about 10 pounds by eating less and counting calories. Then he read a book about fasting to lose weight. He quit eating. Ten days and thirty skipped meals later (not to mention the passed-up between-meal snacks), and 19½ pounds lighter, he decided he had had enough fasting this time around. He was satisfied with his weight loss. So he started eating again. But instead of following refeeding rules, Ziegler took as his first meal a bowl of creamed onion soup, milk, crackers and cheese, a handful of popcorn, and "a bite of my wife's Italian submarine" sandwich.

Ziegler felt fine for a while. But four hours later, during the middle of the night, Ziegler had a rude awakening, and it was painful. He braved the cramps, spasms, and aches for about three hours. Then, at four in the morning, he headed for the hospital. "They gave me some Maalox," Ziegler says, "and I stayed there for about an hour. Then the hospital called my doctor." When the pain let up a little more, Ziegler got back into his car and drove to his doctor's office.

"My doctor said it was a stupid thing to do—both fasting and eating that way after a long fast," Ziegler says. The doctor gave Ziegler a bottle of Maalox and sent him home.

Once Ziegler had eaten the way he did, nothing really could be done to ease the pain. He had already made two big mistakes that could not be undone: he had not consulted a doctor before starting his fast, and he had not allowed his body to readjust to eating by beginning with easy-to-digest foods. The first violation could have resulted in serious consequences; the second brings usually temporary, albeit very painful, discomfort. Ziegler had read the rules. "But I just thought it couldn't happen to me that way," he says, "I thought that only happened to the other guy. You know the syndrome." As Ziegler found out, fasting is no time for the cavalier "rules are made to be broken" attitude. When you fast, you don't just stop eating.

TWO UNBREAKABLE RULES

The two most important rules have already been mentioned, but it will do no harm to repeat them. First, if you have been fasting for more than a few days and you begin to get hungry again—real hunger, not a twinge set off after sitting through four cake, candy, and cookie commercials on television—start eating again. With the return of hunger, your body is warning you that it has used up most of your stored nourishment. To keep alive, the body must now increase mobilization of essential protein tissues, a deathly dangerous prospect. As a corollary to rule one, if you have fasted for four or five days and hunger has never disappeared, stop fasting. For some reason that only a doctor can diagnose, your metabolism may not have adapted to the fasting mode.

Second, consult your doctor before beginning a fast of more than a day or two. Although you believe you are healthy, you may have latent physical conditions, such as a tendency toward diabetes or gout, or an irregular heartbeat, that could preclude your fasting. If you are already seeing a doctor regularly for an illness or any physical condition, you must ask permission before you fast. Some persons should never fast because they have chronic ailments. If you have a liver, kidney, heart, or blood disease, you cannot fast. If you have gout or diabetes, you cannot fast. If you have hypoglycemia, you may be able to fast, but only with medical supervision. Pregnant women should not fast, because they may harm the developing baby. Women who are nursing should not fast. Children generally should not fast. There are many other diseases or conditions that contraindicate fasting, to use the words of one doctor. But listing them would circumvent the purpose of rule two. The point is that someone who wants to fast for any long period of time should see a physician first. The potential harm to your health looms large in fasting, if only because you may not be aware of physical conditions or combinations of several factors that would make fasting inadvisable for you.

There is a second reason for consulting a doctor. Some drugs you may be using should not be taken during a fast. Aspirin and arthritis medication, for example, should not be taken on an empty stomach. This whole question—how the body reacts to drugs during a fast—needs much more study, doctors admit. Because the body is not getting outside nourishment and because some body functions have stopped, slowed down, or changed, it may need increased doses of some drugs and decreased portions of others. A doctor can usually tell you what to do about dosage, which drugs your body will tolerate during a fast, and which may cause adverse reactions.

Almost every fasting advocate would agree on the two basic rules just mentioned. They are the two absolutes. But other rules, or interpretations of them, are not so cast in concrete. Many superstitions, half-truths, and seat-of-the-pants instincts surround the practice. This is not to say they are wrong. But if you read about fasting in various sources, you will find conflicting precepts: stay in bed versus increase exercise, take an enema versus don't use one, drink mineral water versus drink distilled water. There are at least two reasons for these differences of opinion: first, all bodies don't perform in exactly the same way and, second, many fasting advocates do not abide by scientific fact and analysis. The medical world has examined the use of fasting only in connection with weight reduction. It has only considered one value of fasting. Researchers have not addressed its use as a therapy, nor have they acknowledged a need for the body to be cleansed of the toxins that fasting supposedly removes.

PUTTING METHOD IN THIS MADNESS

Nevertheless, here are some rules and suggestions for newcomers to fasting. There are two ways to begin a fast: cold turkey or after a wind-down. Those who go cold turkey just quit eating, often after dinner one evening. Others find it easier to start fasting after breakfast in the morning, spacing the first big hunger hurdle during the night, after they have gone to sleep. If you want to try fasting cold turkey, which time you plan to start depends on your usual hunger patterns. If you usually eat a big breakfast, the latter path would probably be best for you. If you are not usually very hungry in the morning anyway, the former would probably be your choice.

If you feel you have to ease into fasting, try winding down with a prefast diet. For the three days before you want to start fasting, eat successively less.

"When I want to fast, I eat a 1,000-calorie diet one day, only fruits and nuts on the second day, and only juice on the day before," says one veteran faster. "By the fourth day, it's easy to eat nothing." The wind-down is generally for people who have will-power, however. Many people find that even one bite of food makes them hungry all day. These people would only prolong the days of hunger by winding down. If you are one of them, go the cold turkey route.

In any case, you will probably find it most difficult to fast after a day of feasting. If you have had a big breakfast and lunch, followed by dinner at a four-star restaurant and a night of partying, don't try to fast the next day unless you have a will of steel. Your body had to work overtime to process all the food you ate yesterday. It is geared up for a similar day with plenty of food and drink. It is probably best to eat a normal day's food before stopping eating altogether.

By the way, whether you go the cold turkey or wind-down route, many fasters suggest that you eat more than your normal share of raw foods and roughage before you fast. This will help your body eliminate its wastes without difficulty after you stop eating. Many fasting practitioners insist that enemas are necessary to aid the cleansing process. In most cases, however, they are not. The body generally takes good care of itself. Many fasters continue to have bowel movements throughout a fast; others stop after the first few days.

During the fast, hunger will dissipate (mostly) if you sip water all day, as your body requires it. As previously mentioned in the physiology chapter, there is no need to force down large quantities of water. Many fasters or doctors recommend at least 2 quarts (eight regular glasses) of water each day. The kidneys do need a certain amount of water to function properly and to avoid being damaged. But your body will usually tell you how much it requires; follow its signals and you cannot go wrong.

What kind of water? This is another bone of contention among fasting proponents. Many insist that to purify your body you must drink only distilled water. Others suggest that mineral or spring water will supply your body with needed minerals; this is a help, because minerals are normally supplied by food. Others say tap water serves the same purpose because, depending on location, it usually contains minerals, too. Actually, this is a false issue. It really does not matter very much. Drink whatever water you wish. There is no real cause for going out to spend two dollars for a bottle of imported mineral water.

On a true, pure fast, you should drink nothing but water. But many fasters want to drink black coffee, tea, and diet soft drinks. If you are fasting to clean your body from food additives, dyes, and other chemicals, you will defeat that purpose by drinking these beverages. But if you are fasting to lose weight, and for only that reason, go ahead and drink them. It will not slow the weight loss, although it may make you feel hungry.

If possible, you should drink your water at something close to room temperature. Since the body is functioning at a lower metabolism rate, the body's temperature has dropped slightly. It is more sensitive to cold. A cold glass of water could shock the body and give you shivers for a while. But if the thermometer reads 90° F., it is unlikely that your body would be unable to recuperate from a slight chill. Go ahead and have an ice cube in your glass.

More than a glass of cold water can give you the chills. If you are in a season and climate where cold temperatures are the order of the day, take care to keep warm. Many fasting spas strongly encourage sunbathing. The value lies not only in the sun's function as a provider of cheek color and vitamin D, but also because it keeps the body warm.

As happens elsewhere, good intentions can lead one astray, and trying to keep warm can lead a novice faster to another pitfall: taking hot baths, long showers, saunas, or steam baths. Your blood pressure already has decreased, and it can drop even further if you take long baths. This can lead to dizziness or blackout spells.

The blood pressure problem can assert itself in another way. If you bound out of bed in the morning, you may find yourself dizzy, too. Changes in body position require a change in blood pressure. After several days of fasting, the adaptive response of blood pressure has slowed down. This sluggishness can make you feel faint or dizzy if you make a sudden move. However, this problem is easy to avoid. When moving from lying to standing positions or when you bend over to pick something up, just slow down your movements to give your body time to adjust. If you do get dizzy because you moved too quickly, sit or stand in the second position, waiting until the body adjusts.

Actually, few changes in daily life are demanded of a faster. Although many of those who proselytize about fasting for its therapeutic value insist that you remain in bed during a fast, this is nonsense for any fast that you can undertake without medical supervision. You can go to work, clean house, garden, and shop as you normally would and, if you have the willpower, you can go to any party or social event that you care to attend.

What about exercise? This is another hot spot where opinions vary widely, from those who insist that none be undertaken to those who talk of fasters running the Boston marathon. In general, the best guide to follow is your body's tolerance for exercise and its past experience with it. In other words, if you have been following a regular routine of exercise, you can keep it up during a fast. But don't start a new exhaustive regimen. You may find yourself passing out. Exercise always gets the body working to mobilize fat tissue, however, and that satisfies hunger. So if you have been exercising and you keep it up during a fast, you may find yourself less hungry than a sedentary faster. If you have not been exercising regularly, at least try a long walk or some other nonstrenuous exercise.

WHEN YOU START EATING AGAIN

That should take care of what you do during the fast; ending one is another matter. Just as starting to fast looks simple, ending one looks even simpler. But it is not, and that is where Lou Ziegler got into trouble at the beginning of this chapter. You cannot just start eating again.

Even if your fast has lasted only a day or two, your body has gotten out of the habit of digesting food. It has cut back the production of digestive enzymes, and it cannot resume full production immediately. If you start eating a thick, juicy steak, an ice cream cone or a fast-food doubleburger, you will find yourself suffering the severe indigestion pains that drove Lou Ziegler to the emergency room. Even if you do not go that far, you may be spending an unusual amount of time in the bathroom, waiting out a long spell of stomach cramps and diarrhea.

A refeeding period gives your body time to get used to digesting food again. If you want to change your eating habits, it also allows you to replace bad old routines with new healthy ones. The length depends on how long you fasted—one day of refeeding for every two or three fast days.

The idea behind refeeding, then, is to start with easy-to-digest food, a bland diet. Most fasters begin with juice, often diluted orange juice. Orange juice is loaded with potassium, an essential mineral the body has been missing during the fast. Take regular-strength orange, grapefruit, or apple juice and mix it with water. Many fasters suggest equal amounts of juice and water, but others find that too weak and use half as much water. Do whichever your taste prefers. During the first day after a fast of a week or more, you should probably stick only with juices. Sip several glasses of juice during the day. If you must have something else, have clear vegetable soup, a half of a grapefruit, or a bit of plain, unsweetened yogurt, mixed, if you wish, with a bit of grated fruit. Stay away from anything that is high in fat; a fat load in refeeding can precipitate diarrhea or a gallbladder attack.

After the first day, you can gradually increase the amount of solid food that you eat. On the first day of eating solids, again choose low-fat foods: a baked apple, a mashed banana or poached pear, yogurt, cooked rice, ricotta or cottage cheese, or vegetable soups. Then move on to raw carrots, cabbage and tomatoes, grapes, baked or boiled potatoes, low-fat cheeses, and so on. When you come to the end of your refeeding, as calculated by the length of your fast, you can resume eating whatever you wish. Through it all, you will help avoid indigestion by taking many small meals instead of three large ones, by eating slowly, and by chewing food thoroughly.

As you break the fast, particularly if you gave up food to lose weight and want to avoid a demoralizing weight gain disproportionate to the food you are consuming, avoid all salt. It will make your body retain water and the reading on the scale will climb back up very quickly. Many processed and canned foods such as soups contain high amounts of salt, so you would want to avoid them.

All right, so you have gone through a two-week fast and shed 18 pounds. But six weeks later you have already regained more than half the loss. Can you fast again? Yes, but not immediately. Generally, the body cannot accommodate repeated fasting without sufficient time in between. Doctors suggest waiting at least three months between fasts of more than one week and six months to one year between fasts of two to three weeks. Otherwise, cumulative effects can mount; without your knowledge, you may be doing more harm than occurs during a once-only fast or sufficiently spaced fasts.

However, it may be more beneficial, not to say easier, for you to embark on several shorter fasts instead of one prolonged one. This is especially true if you just want to clean your body of food additives—since that takes at most only a couple of days—or if you fast to maintain your weight. A one-day fast can occur once a week; you can go on a two- or three-day fast once a month.

Remember that at any time during the fast, if anything unusual occurs, see your doctor and stop fasting. The chances of anything happening are small, but you should not continue the fast if you are experiencing severe stomachaches, nausea and vomiting, prolonged headaches, an irregular heartbeat, faintness, dizziness, or any severe pain.

For your convenience, the rules are repeated here without the long explanations.

1. Start eating again when true hunger returns.
2. Consult your doctor before starting a fast.
3. Take no drugs during a fast without first getting a doctor's permission.
4. If necessary, ease into a fast with a preparatory diet.
5. Whether or not you prepare to fast with a special diet, try to help your body eliminate wastes by eating roughage before you fast. There is usually no need to take an enema.
6. Drink as much water, preferably at room temperature, as your body requires.
7. Keep warm.
8. Avoid long baths and showers and all steam and sauna baths.
9. Move slowly when changing positions from lying to sitting or standing or when bending over.
10. Exercise as you would in your normal everyday life.
11. Let your body readjust to food by going through a refeeding period during which you eat only bland, low-fat foods.
12. Fast only at intervals long enough to give your body a chance to replace all the protein it lost and regain strength.
13. See your doctor if anything out of the ordinary happens to your body during a fast.

THE HAPPY ENDING

What happened to Lou Ziegler, the hapless reporter who started this chapter? Ziegler wrote his story, "The Crash Diet That Crashed," for his newspaper, after talking with two more doctors. He gained back about 10 pounds. But fasting did not, so to speak, leave a bad taste in his mouth. He has tried it again and his weight is down to 180 pounds. "Now I try to fast one day a week to maintain my weight. I usually fast on Monday, and it takes off the weight I may have put on over the weekend. I don't mind it at all," he says. "You just have to know how to use it."

10
fasting farms

YOU HAVE MADE the decision to fast, but your body is rebelling against your mind's decision. You are one of the many people who cannot turn off their appetites at will. Even enthusiastic fasters sometimes have difficulties. "There are days when a fast just won't work," says one of them. "You're just not prepared for it. But if I'm feeling good about fasting, I can watch other people eat and it doesn't bother me a bit. It was quite something to discover that I can enjoy going to the movies without eating popcorn."

You try again. This time you have gotten yourself all psyched up to do it; you go all the way to nine o'clock at night, but you just cannot stand it anymore. Your spouse, your child, a roommate, a friend, maybe even a person on television is munching on something and you cannot watch any longer. Your willpower goes to pieces.

You are not alone. Many people cannot fast with so many external stimuli turning on their appetites and breaking their resolve. In fact, many people do not realize how much their lives center around eating and food until they try to fast. If you are one of those who cannot fast alone, you can still try it, but you will have to put out some money to do it.

Unless you are massively obese and under a doctor's orders to fast, a hospital will probably not take you in merely to fast. But you can go to one of the many fasting farms (the owners usually object to that term) around the country. They are special spas, not like the twelve-hundred-dollar-a-week beauty spas you may have heard about. Most are small, comparatively spartan places that do not pamper their customers.

Generally there are two kinds of fasting farms—those whose prime reason for being is weight reduction and those that concentrate on health. The latter are often run by natural hygienists, often members of the American Natural Hygiene Society.

Both categories have reputable as well as shoddy outfits. Before you decide to go, ask a lot of questions. If possible, try to talk with people who have been there. Many of these spas are located in Florida and California in order to capitalize on the warm weather and sun, but some do exist in New York, Canada, and Texas. (Europeans support fasting spas, too—ask your travel agent.) There may be more but, because there is no central information or trade association, there is no comprehensive list of them. Many advertise in city or health magazines or newspapers, so you might try checking there.

The weight-reduction spas usually exist in an upbeat atmosphere. Customers can attend classes in nutrition, diet, and exercise. They can learn yoga and get a massage. Game rooms—with playing cards, backgammon, and so on—and swimming pools abound. Some offer more. New Image, a new spa in Toronto, brings in fashion consultants, hairdressers, cosmeticians, and arts and crafts teachers. Doctors usually stop in periodically for a visit.

Most spas require clients to spend a minimum amount of time. Drydock, located in Quantico, Virginia, asks the least—a minimum of three days at thirty-five dollars a day. But it recommends a seven-day stay that would include a three-day total fast followed by four days on a modified fast. Even though Drydock's ad beckons fasters with a line reading, "If you can't fast at home, come fast at Drydock," it will not allow customers to undertake a total fast for more than three days. New Image requires a seven-day stay at $295 for the first week and $275 for the second. Guests there spend the entire time on a water fast, which results in an average loss of 10 to 20 pounds, respectively, over the one- or two-week periods. They can also pay an additional $150 to take part in an eight-week followup program in which members meet once weekly to discuss the fast, get help in nutrition and meal planning, and learn low-calorie cooking.

The natural hygiene spas concentrate on spreading the word about their health philosophy, although the pitch is very low-key. Most have no schedules; guests are free to do what they wish with their time. But they are more regimented—no smoking, for example.

Located outside of San Antonio, Texas, Dr. Shelton's Health School has supervised fasts since 1928. Herbert Shelton wrote many books about fasting and natural hygiene and was one of the prime movers in establishing the American Natural Hygiene Society. He called his place a health school, not a spa, because he wanted it to teach all guests natural hygiene. "Where health is built . . . not bought" is the school's motto. For between twenty-four and thirty dollars a day, guests can fast as they learn about unprocessed and unrefined foods, exercise, sunshine, and fresh air at lectures and by listening to tape recordings. They cannot leave the school grounds, and exercise other than walking is discouraged. "For a longer period of time we have had them rest instead of exercising," says a promotional brochure, "and we are convinced that those who rest fare better. They recover health faster and their body stores up more nerve energy than those who exercise while fasting." Shelton's offers no cures to ill guests, but many people who come are sick. A chiropractor is in charge.

Those who don't come to get well at natural hygiene spas usually come to vacation, to rest, and sometimes to lose weight. Most are white, middle-class people, with a higher proportion of women than men. In age, the majority is either oldish—above fifty years of age—or relatively young—twenties. The spas try to create an environment of health and rest. Many do not permit television watching, and many suggest an early afternoon siesta. Facilities vary, but guests usually dress casually, listen to lectures and discussions, and spend the rest of their time sunbathing, reading, swimming, taking exercise classes, and resting. A few have tennis or boating facilities. Not everyone fasts, however, and you may be tempted on occasion by someone eating fruits, vegetables, and nuts.

Among the general public, Pawling Health Manor in Hyde Park, New York, is probably the most well known of the fasting farms. James Earl Jones, Norman Mailer, Pete Hammill, Shirley MacLaine, and many other famous people are among the 25,000 who have come to this retreat 100 miles north of New York City in the twenty years of its existence. The director, Robert R. Gross, advises his customers to see a doctor before coming to stay (for a minimum of a week). Gross charges at least $155 for the one-week stay; rates vary according to accommodations. Most people, he says, stay longer than a week. Obese customers have remained as long as four months.

Gross, a physiochemist who is a member of the American Natural Hygiene Society, offers no frills. People come to lose weight, either by total fasting or by a low-calorie modified fast, and that is what they do. They can listen to records, read books about health, take trips to nearby historic sites or to the movies in a nearby town, play cards, watch television, take walks, or just sleep. There is a gymnasium, but there are no yoga classes, exercise sessions, swimming pool, or tennis courts. Guests are essentially on their own, except for a daily pulse check. Guests can, of course, seek out advice from Gross and his staff, but there is little pushiness on their part. Typically, guests arrive on Sunday and fast totally until Friday, when they are given orange juice (or another kind) at lunch and at dinner. Before they leave on Saturday, they eat fruit —grapefruit or a baked apple, for example. They continue refeeding on their own at home.

That is the sort of schedule, instruction, and activity you can expect at most fasting farms. Other guests will offer the moral support you may need to fast; like many diets, fasting is easier if you have someone with whom to commiserate. Gross's motto is also helpful to remember, whether or not you visit a fasting farm: "Fifteen minutes at a time." If you approach it that way, he says, you can keep a fast.

epilog

"Fasting is medicine."

—ST. JOHN CHRYSOSTOM,
FOURTH CENTURY.

"Say, can you fast? Your stomachs are too young.
And abstinence engenders maladies."

—WILLIAM SHAKESPEARE, SIXTEENTH CENTURY.

THE TWO SPEAKERS lived in different times and different places, but that does not matter. As we have seen, fasting did not fall out of favor, then or now. The difference of opinion about fasting has probably always existed. Voluntary fasting has been controversial from its beginnings. Since it became popular, so many claims have been made about fasting that it could be nothing but disputatious, particularly with regard to its health benefits.

Even in religion, fasting has its boosters and detractors. Some clergymen would have you believe that fasting is essential for salvation, but Martin Luther and philosopher Immanuel Kant are among those who wrote against it. "One good deed is better than three days of fasting," a Japanese proverb says. As a measure of protest, fasting has seen many successes and many more failures.

Today, most newcomers come to fasting, however, not for religious and protest reasons, but for diet or health motives. If Americans no longer believe that a fountain of youth exists, many are at least searching for a fountain of health as a means to a longer life. We have all heard perhaps the healthicst people in the world—the Russian residents of areas in the Caucasus mountains, of Yukatia in Siberia, and of the Poltaya district in the Ukraine, who often lead active lives beyond the age of 100 and even 150 years—credit their way of life, their eating and drinking habits, and their high participation in physical activity as the reason for their longevity. We have seen other evidence that a better lifestyle can improve health, and doctors now expect interest in the control of personal habits to increase. Study after study has demonstrated that eating habits should be a major source of concern. Then, last year, a survey showed that 98 percent of the respondents believed that overeating was a major barrier to improved nutrition and thus to a better way of life. Typically, many Americans sought out the simplest, fastest solution to overeating —a fast, they thought, could be the quick fix every now and then.

Fasting has demonstrable and theoretical benefits with regard to health, weight control, body cleansing, and discipline, as we have seen. It has its uses. But it will not cure you of any illness. The old adage about starving a fever does not hold water, nor is it valid for any other disease. The human body often demands less food when it is ailing, but the sick person should eat as much as he or she can tolerate as a means to regain strength. This is particularly evident when you consider that a fever will elevate the metabolism rate, making the body burn more than its usual number of calories and making it dip into lean muscle tissues earlier than would be expected.

Some people should never fast, those with heart or liver disease, for example. Children should not fast; the lack of adequate calories can stunt growth. No studies of fasting have proven this, but medical researchers extrapolate from knowledge that other forms of malnutrition retard the physical and even mental development of children in poor countries.

If you wish, you can probably fast for a day or two by yourself, but you should consult a doctor first. The medical world does not have a ready answer to charges that physicians do not know enough about nutrition and fasting to deserve consultation. Many doctors are so utterly opposed to it that they will not comment beyond saying that they are against fasting in any way, shape, or form. If your doctor is one of those, find another before you fast. And many doctors, too, are getting more interested in nutrition. The American Medical Association reports that nutrition courses at medical schools are becoming more popular. According to a 1976 survey, almost 20 percent of the 114 schools now require students to take a nutrition course. Another 70 percent of medical schools offer it as an elective, and 95 percent include instruction in basic nutrition in other required courses. This does not mean that your doctor has a working knowledge of nutrition or fasting, nor does it signify that doctors are keeping up with the subject once they graduate from medical school. But it is an improvement.

If you plan to fast for longer than a few days, you should consult your doctor; in the case of a fast longer than seven to ten days, a hospital stay is advisable.

Fasting can be a successful dieting routine if the faster also relearns good eating and activity habits. Fasting can reduce dependence on food and help an overweight person discover what true hunger feels like. Doctors generally feel that its use should be restricted to obese people who can be monitored during the fast's duration; for others, they question the dangers associated with the loss of lean tissue and bone matter, among other concerns. As a diet, studies show that success in losing and maintaining the loss is independent of sex, age, length of obesity, level of physical activity, and other factors. It appears that attitude may be the key to success. Fasting one day a week has also been shown to be a good weight maintenance device. For the ordinary person, this is probably fasting's most effective use.

In short, fasting does not do all that its advocates claim. There may be a place for it in some people's way of living, but it will probably not be a prominent one. In any case, it is always better to eat a well-balanced, moderate diet and to practice good living habits to ensure good health. There are no shortcuts to that goal.

bibliography

Allen, Thomas H., Ph.D., and Musgrave, Paul W., M.D. "Gross Composition of Weight Loss in Obese Men on a 400-Calorie Diet." *The American Journal of Clinical Nutrition* (January 1971).

Ashe, Geoffrey. *Gandhi*. New York: Stein and Day, 1968.

Barnard, D.L., et al. "Changes in Body Composition Produced by Prolonged Total Starvation and Refeeding." *Metabolism* (July 1969).

Benoit, Frederick L., Martin, Robert L., and Walter, Raymond H. "Changes in Body Composition During Weight Reduction in Obesity." *Annals of Internal Medicine* (October 1965).

The Catholic University of America. *New Catholic Encyclopedia*. New York: McGraw-Hill, 1967.

Clark, Blake. "A Sure, Swift Way to Take Off Weight." *Reader's Digest* (November 1962).

Consolazio, C. Frank, et al. "Metabolic Aspects of Calorie Restriction: Nitrogen and Mineral Balances and Vitamin Excretion." *The American Journal of Clinical Nutrition* (August 1968).

DeVries, Arnold. *Therapeutic Fasting*. Greene, Iowa: Chandler Book Co., 1963.

DeWitt, Karen. "Fasting." *The Washington Post* (2 August 1977).

Dukes, Sir Paul. *The Yoga of Health, Youth and Joy*. New York: Harper & Brothers, 1960.

Encyclopedia Judaica. New York: Macmillan, 1971.

Epstein, Edward Jay. "Good News From Mr. Bad News." *New York* (9 August 1976).

Evans, Ivor H. *Brewer's Dictionary of Phrase and Fable*. Rev. ed. New York: Harper & Row, 1970.

Fairweather, Eugene R. *The Meaning and Message of Lent*. New York: Harper & Brothers, 1962.

Gandhi, Mohandas K. *Letters to a Disciple*. New York: Harper & Brothers, 1950.

Gibb, H.A.R., and Kramers, J.H. *Shorter Encyclopedia of Islam*. Ithaca, N.Y.: Cornell University Press, 1953.

Goldstein, Jack. *Triumph Over Disease—By Fasting and Natural Diet*. New York: Arco Publishing, 1977.

Goodhart, Robert S., and Shils, Maurice E., eds. *Modern Nutrition in Health and Disease*. 5th ed. Philadelphia: Lea & Febiger, 1973.

Goodman, Felicitas D., Henney, Jeannette H., and Pressel, Esther. *Trance, Healing, and Hallucination—Three Field Studies in Religious Experience*. New York: John Wiley & Sons, 1974.

Gray, Louis Herbert, A.M., Ph.D., ed. *The Mythology of All Races*. New York: Cooper Square Publishers, 1964.

Gregory, Dick, with James R. McGraw. *Up From Nigger*. New York: Stein and Day, 1976.

Harris, Leon. *Upton Sinclair—American Rebel*. New York: Thomas Y. Crowell, 1975.

Hendrickson, Bill. "Supervised Liquid-Protein Diet Shows Promise in Treating Obesity, Despite Recent Problems." *The Wall Street Journal* (17 November 1977).

Hoffman, Norman S. *A New World of Health*. New York: McGraw-Hill, 1977.

Howard, Jane. "How I Lost 14 Pounds in a Week." *Family Circle* (October 1974).

Hughes, Thomas Patrick. *A Dictionary of Islam*. London: W.H. Allen, 1935.

"Hunger Strikers: A Medical Problem." *Medical World News* (1 December 1975).

Kent, Rosemary. "Fasting Is In." *Cosmopolitan* (August 1976).

Kremer, William F., M.D., and Kremer, Laura, M.D. *The Doctors' Metabolic Diet*. New York: Crown, 1975.

Lame Deer, John Fire, and Richard Ardoes. *Lame Deer, Seeker of Visions*. New York: Simon and Schuster, 1972.

Mencken, H.L., ed. *A New Dictionary of Quotations*. New York: Alfred A. Knopf, 1977.

Radin, Paul, Ph.D. *The Story of the American Indian*. New York: Liveright Publishing, 1944.

Reed, Roy. "Fast by Three Men Forces Dublin to Eat Crow." *The New York Times* (4 May 1978).

Renou, Louis, ed. *Hinduism*. New York: George Braziller, 1962.

"Risk Analysis: It Can Help People Change Their Ways." *Medical World News* (4 November 1977).

Roberts, Nancy. *The Yoga Thing*. New York: Hawthorn Books, 1973.

Robinson, Corinne H., M.S., R.D. *Normal and Therapeutic Nutrition*, 14th ed. New York: Macmillan, 1972.

Rosten, Leo. *Treasury of Jewish Quotations*. New York: Bantam Books, 1977.

Shelton, Herbert M. *Fasting for Renewal of Life*. Chicago: Natural Hygiene Press, 1974.

Terrell, John Upton. *Sioux Trail*. New York: McGraw-Hill, 1974.

The Jewish Encyclopedia. New York: Funk and Wagnalls, 1906.

The New English Bible. England: The Oxford University Press and The Cambridge University Press, 1961.

Thomson, T.J., Runcie, J., and Miller, V. "Treatment of Obesity by Total Fasting for Up to 249 Days." *The Lancet* (5 November 1966).

"To Fast or Not to Fast." *America* (31 March 1962).

Toynbee, Arnold. *A Study of History*. Oxford: The Oxford University Press, 1972.

Troebst, Cord Christian. *The Art of Survival*. Garden City, N.Y.: Doubleday, 1965.

Warren, William N. *History of the Ojibway Nation*. Minneapolis: Ross & Haines, 1970.

Weinsier, Roland L., M.D. "Fasting—A Review with Emphasis on the Electrolytes." *The American Journal of Medicine* (February 1971).

Wolfe, Tom. "The 'Me' Decade." *New York* (23 August 1976).

Young, Vernon R., and Scrimshaw, Nevin S. "The Physiology of Starvation." *Scientific American* (October 1971).

Zimmer, Heinrich. *Philosophies of India*. New York: Pantheon Books, 1951.

index

Absolute, union with the, 39, 40
American Indians, 19–23
American Medical Association, 60, 110
American Natural Hygiene Society, 55–61 *passim*, 106, 108

Baader-Meinhof gang, 48
bariatrics, 10, 13
Blackburn, Dr. George L., 78
Buddhism, 15, 40–41: *see also* Hinduism
Busk ceremony, 19–20

Cahill, Dr. George F., Jr., 88
catabolism, 85, 91
Catholics: see Eastern Catholics; Roman Catholics
celebrity fasters, 3, 43
Celtic myths, 20
Chibcha Indians, 19
children, 97, 110
China: see Taoism; Lao Tzu
cholesterol, 13, 14
Christians,35–38

Daniel, Book of (Bible), 32
death from fasting, 4: liquid protein diet deaths, 80–81
demons, casting out, 19
Didache (early Christian writing), 37
diet, 13–14, 69–81 *passim*: and modified fasts, 77–81; designing a diet for fasters, 78
diseases and disorders, 56–81 *passim*
Doctor Shelton's Health School (fasting spa), 107
doctors, 60–63, 71–72: opposed to fasting, 84
Dolci, Danilo, 46–47
Drydock (fasting spa), 106

Eastern Catholics, 38
Edison, Thomas A., 55
Eid ul Fitr (festival), 25
Elijah (prophet), 35
Esther, Book of (Bible), 31

fast day, 38, 49, 50
fasting: popularity gain, 2; definition of, 4; survival and, 4, 85; as a fad, 7; reasons for, 9; and future, 9–11; renaissance of, 11–12; prosperity and, 12–13; origin of, 17–23 *passim*; water and, 90, 99, 100; how to, 95–103; two major rules, 96–97; newcomers to, 98; ending, 100, 101, 102, 103, 111
fasting farms, 105–108: *see also* fasting spas
fasting spas, 100: *see also* Dr. Shelton's Health School; Drydock; New Image; Pawling Health Manor
Five Pillars of Islam, 30
folklore, 17–24
food: America's love affair with, 1; quantity consumed in America, 2–9, 10; new foods, 10
Food and Drug Administration, U.S., 80

Gandhi, Mohandas K., 43–46 *passim*, 47, 50
Genuth, Dr. Sol, 78
Germany, Nazi, 48–49, 50, 51
glucose, 84, 85, 86, 88
glycogen, 88–89
Goldstein, Jack, 59
Graham, Sylvester, 56
Gregory, Dick, 51–52
guardian spirit, cult of, 23

habits, changing of, 13: eating, 13, 84, 85, 86
Harris, Emily, 50–51
health, 15, 53–67: claims, 63–67; losing weight by fasting, 69–81; body adjustments to fasting, 83–94; ending a fast, 100, 101, 102, 103
Health Robbers, The (book), 61
Hebrews: see Judaism
Hinduism, 15, 38–42 *passim*
Hoffman, Prof. Norman F., 11
Huberman, Mark, 57–60 *passim*
hunger strikes, 47, 48, 49: G. Gordon Liddy, 50; Golda Meir, 50; Dick Gregory, 51–52
hygiene, 55–60, 61–63

India: see Buddhism; Hinduism; Gandhi, Mohandas K.; Nehru, Jawaharlal
Indians, American: see American Indians
IRA (Irish Republican Army), 48
Ireland, 48
Islam, 27–30: *see also* Ramadan

Jesus Christ, 35–38 *passim*
Jews: see Judaism
Jogging: *see* running
Jordan, Henry A., 13
Judaism, 20, 26, 30–35 *passim*: laws of fasting, 33–35

Kafka, Franz, 3
Kant, Emanuel, 109
ketogenesis, 64, 88, 92, 93
Koran, 27–30 *passim*

Lao Tzu, 42
Lent, 38
Liddy, G. Gordon, 43: hunger strike, 50

liquid protein diet, 80: deaths from, 80–81
long fasts, 90–94, 111
Luther, Martin, 109

magic and ritual fasting, 18
Manicheans, 41
Matthew, Book of (Bible), 35, 38
medically supervised fasting, 5
Megillat Ta'amit (tractate of Talmud), 30, 31
modified fasts, 78–81
Meir, Golda, leading a hunger strike, 50
Mormons, 38
Moses, 30, 35
Moslems: see Muslims
Muslims, 27–30, 45–46: *see also* Ramadan
Mythology of All Races (book), cited, 20

National Academy of Science, 87
National Center for Health Statistics, 70
National Heart, Lung and Blood Institute, 14
Nazis, 48–49, 50, 51
Nehru, Jawaharlal, 46
New Image (fasting spa), 106
nutrition, 2, 10

obesity, 5, 9: weight reduction, 14, 69–81 *passim*, 105
Oral Roberts University, suspension of fat students, 70

Pauling, Linus, 15
Pawling Health Manor (fasting spa), 107–108
penance, 27, 36
Pharisees, 36
Pius XII, Pope, 37
Plato, 3
political fasts, 43–52
protein: protein-sparing diet, 78; liquid protein, 80; loss of proteins, 91

Ramadan rites, 25
religion and fasting, 15, 109: *see also* Buddhism; Christians; Hinduism; Islam; Mormons; Muslims; Roman Catholics; Taoism; Zonoastrianism
Roman Catholics, 37–38
running and jogging, 13, 66–67
Running and Being (book), 66

Scientific American (magazine), 88
Shaw, George Bernard, 1
Sheehan, Dr. George A., 66
Shelley, Mary, 47
Sinclair, Upton, 65
Slade, Madeleine, 44
Socrates, 3
Story of the American Indian, The (book), 23
Symbionese Liberation Army, 50–57

Talmud, 30–33 *passim*: *see also* *Megillat Ta'amit*
Taoism, 42
Triumph Over Disease (book), 59

Vindication of the Rights of Women, The (book), 47

weight reduction, 14: modified fasts, 78–81; weight reduction

weight reduction (*cont.*)
spas, 105–108; *see also* obesity, diet
Wollstonecraft, Mary, 47
women (nursing), 97
World War II, and hunger strikes, 47, 48, 49, 50

Yoga, 15, 40
Yoga of Health, Youth and Joy, The, 40
Yom Kippur (Day of Atonement), 25–26

Zoroastrianism, 40–41